WHAT OTHERS SAY ABOUT THIS BOOK...

Most chronic diseases are due to our behaviors, yet many people have a hard time changing their diet and lifestyle. In Healthy Habits, Helpful Friends, *Judd Allen eloquently describes how the support of our loved ones can often make a critically important difference. This book is a passionate call to action, and I highly recommend it.*

> —Dean Ornish, M.D., Founder and President, Preventive Medicine Research Institute, Clinical Professor of Medicine, University of California, San Francisco, and Author, *Love & Survival* and *Dr. Dean Ornish's Program for Reversing Heart Disease*

The peer support approach was very helpful at Union Pacific Railroad. Too often health improvement programs neglect the team and focus exclusively on individual change. Teamwork is central to other successful business practices. Healthy Habits, Helpful Friends *applies this fundamental business strategy toward creating healthier corporate cultures and healthier employees.*

> — Joe Leutzinger, Ph.D., Principal, Health Improvement Solutions and former Director of Health Promotion, Union Pacific Railroad

This groundbreaking book continues the Allen family tradition of addressing the need for cultural support to achieve wellness. Dr. Allen, like his father, the late Dr. Robert Allen, offers a unique and much-needed perspective on how we can work together to bring about lasting and positive change.

> — Don Ardell, Ph.D., Editor, *The Ardell Wellness Report*

Healthy Habits, Helpful Friends *shows us how support from others is key to successful behavior change. It is practically impossible to adopt and maintain healthy behaviors without it.*

> — Steven Aldana, Ph.D., Author, *The Culprit & The Cure* and *The Stop & Go Fast Food Nutrition Guide*

Healthy Habits, Helpful Friends *is a comprehensive resource for health promotion practitioners seeking to build a foundation for cultural change. A 'must have' to provide optimal behavior change interventions and support.*

> — Erica Wandtke, M.A., National Hea
> U.S. Department of Health and Humai

HEALTHY HABITS, HELPFUL FRIENDS

How to Effectively Support Wellness Lifestyle Goals

Judd Allen, Ph.D.

President, Human Resources Institute, LLC

Published by

healthyculture.com

Burlington, Vermont

Healthy Habits, Helpful Friends: How to Effectively Support
Wellness Lifestyle Goals

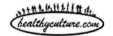

Contact information:

Human Resources Institute, LLC

151 Dunder Road

Burlington, VT 05401 USA

(802) 862-8855

Info@healthyculture.com

www.Healthyculture.com

Quantity purchases of *Healthy Habits, Helpful Friends* are available
for educational, business and community use.

Cover photographs available through Getty Images. The people shown are
models used for illustrative purposes only.

Contents

Acknowledgments

I would like to thank my friends, family, colleagues and clients for their input and enthusiasm for the writing process.

My father, Robert Allen, Ph.D., inspired my interest in supportive cultural environments and wellness. This book is a tribute to his life's work. Until his death, he was my mentor.

Other family members also provided emotional support for my writing efforts. Among them are Anne, Morgan, Peter, Rhonda, Matthew and Robert Allen, as well as Elaine and Bob Smith and Mary and Marvin Sochet.

I'm grateful to my wellness buddies Rick Blount, Jonathan Sands, Rick Hubbard, Emina Burak, Fred Cohen, Jim Carmen, James Dingley, David Means and Clay Warren. These people have shown me the power of peer support in my own life.

Jack Travis, Meryn Callander, Victoria Beliveau, Joe Leutzinger, Feyedra Matthes and Gabe Cohen offered great editorial assistance.

Thanks to my colleagues Troy Adams, Steve Aldana, Carol Ardell, Don Ardell, Bill Baun, Marybeth Baun, Craig Becker, Larry Chapman, Dee Edington, Dennis Elsenrath, David Gobble, Ken Holtyn, Bill Hettler, David Hunnicutt, Michael O'Donnell, Gillian Pieper, Kay Ryan and Elaine Sullivan. These wellness experts have been particularly helpful in making sure my concept of peer support is both based in good science and practical.

Thanks also to the National Wellness Institute, Wellness Councils of America, Health Improvement Solutions, the Institute for Health and Productivity Management and the American Journal of Health Promotion, as well as the many businesses, communities and organizations that have embraced and tested the peer support concepts.

About the Author

Judd Allen earned his Ph.D. in community psychology from New York University. He is President of the Human Resources Institute (also known as Healthyculture.com), a research, publishing and consulting firm that focuses on the creation of supportive cultural environments. Dr. Allen serves on the editorial board of the *American Journal of Health Promotion* and is on the board of directors of the National Wellness Institute and a trustee of Perhaps Kids Meeting Kids Can Make a Difference. He has taught on the faculties of Nebraska Methodist College, Cornell University Medical College and Johnson State College. Dr. Allen moderates four culture change training sites: www.changeculture.com, www.wellnessmentoring.com, www.leadwellness.com, and www.healthyworkclimate.com. Dr. Allen was a senior research analyst at Memorial Sloan-Kettering Cancer Center and has served on the Vermont Governor's Council for Physical Fitness and Sports.

He loves to travel, exercise and play with friends and family. Dr. Allen has completed more than 20 consecutive New York City Marathons as well as Ironman distance triathlons and long-distance cross-country ski races. He lives in Burlington, Vermont, with his wife and daughter.

A Call to Kindness

This book is written for those seeking to help a friend, family member, neighbor or coworker achieve personal lifestyle improvement goals. The wellness goal could be anything that involves day-to-day behavior, including managing stress, maintaining positive relationships, becoming physically active, eating healthier, stopping smoking and controlling alcohol and other substance abuse. The wellness goal could be motivated by any number of factors, including the need to manage a disability or illness, eliminate health risks, increase personal performance or become more socially responsible; or the wish to look better, feel great and enjoy a higher quality of life.

For this book to be of use, your offer of assistance should be heartfelt. You must be open to being as helpful as possible, but you need not compromise your own well-being. You must be willing to suspend your criticism and accept your peer's change goal. You must be open to learning afresh the challenges of achieving a behavior change. You must also understand that your own skills and experiences are important, but your peer will have to find her own best approach to change. If you are not in a good position to provide support at this time, your kindest option would be to find someone willing and able to offer such support.

For this book to be most relevant, your peer should be actively pursuing a new lifestyle practice and open to your help.

This is not a book about why people should make a change, and it does not offer strategies for convincing people why they should change. Instead, this book is for helping people succeed at freely chosen healthy lifestyle goals.

Healthy Habits, Helpful Friends is about increasing the quality and quantity of peer support. It draws upon the collective wisdom of psychology, sociology, anthropology and health promotion to expand your capacity to help with behavior change. This book is based on the lessons learned from Wellness Mentor® programs in business, school, health-care, spa and community settings (further information at www.wellnessmentor.net). *Healthy Habits, Helpful Friends* features six primary support techniques that go far beyond the typical help offered by peers:

1. **Setting Goals.** The focus is on clarifying wellness goals, exploring related scientific knowledge and tailoring personal goals. Both short- and long-term goals are set so they are compatible with the likely behavior change process.

2. **Identifying Role Models.** The focus is on finding someone who has achieved similar wellness goals under similar circumstances. Such a role model would be interviewed to learn more about what worked, what challenges were overcome and other tips that might be useful.

3. **Eliminating Barriers to Change.** Potential physical and psychological barriers are identified. Strategies are developed for breaking down barriers and to overcome them. The approach to barriers is positive with an emphasis on existing strengths and finding the resources needed for success.

4. **Locating Supportive Environments.** Physical and social environments (at work, at home and in the community) are examined to determine how they support or undermine success. Strategies are developed for limiting contact with less-supportive environments and increasing contact with environments that better support wellness goals.

5. **Working through Relapse.** No one wants to get off track and fail to achieve desired behavior change. Game plans are developed for avoiding high-risk situations and for handling a relapse. As a result, the changer will be in a position to learn from these experiences and to make appropriate adjustments.

6. **Celebrating Success.** Most successes go unrecognized. This is unfortunate because it is a missed opportunity for some fun and because rewards reinforce behavior change. You and your peer will identify many occasions to celebrate as well as determine the most meaningful way to make successes count.

Browse the book and pick those strategies that you think are most beneficial and timely. These pages are filled with discussions of best practices, questions, stories and checklists that are meant to stimulate careful consideration of the options. I encourage you and your peer to read through the peer support stories and checklists at the end of each chapter. This is not a recipe book with a one-size-fits-all approach. You and your peer must put your thoughts together to come up with the best solutions given your peer's unique goals and circumstances. Many of these ideas will require patience, perseverance and a trial-and-error approach. By working together, you will dramatically increase the likelihood for lasting and positive behavior change. Your support can lighten the load of difficult change and actually make the change process enjoyable.

Your offer to assist is a tremendous gift. If you fortify your peer support efforts with some of the techniques explained on the following pages, I am confident that your kindness and understanding can make a substantial difference.

To your health,
Judd
Burlington, Vermont

Chapter 1

Building the Foundation for Peer Support

This chapter examines some of the possibilities for organizing your peer support efforts. It will help you to better understand and explain your peer support role. Building a good foundation includes addressing such topics as confidentiality, follow-up, and how your voluntary support fits with that offered by health and wellness professionals. A good foundation enhances trust and openness. Clarity about your approach will make your efforts more effective.

Many People Try to Change without Adequate Support

When it comes to trying to achieve healthier habits, no one should feel alone. Each year approximately 80 percent of the adults in North America attempt to lose weight, manage stress, become more physically active, stop smoking or change another behavior. These change attempts are motivated by a wide range of wellness goals, including the desire to prevent illness, heal, improve performance or achieve a better quality of life. The desires for self-improvement and self-preservation, combined with the ready availability of information on the benefits of healthy practices, appear to be making wellness-related behavior change attempts a common phenomenon. Such change efforts are essential to our own wellness and to the health and well-being of those we care deeply about.

The fact that we are attempting health behavior changes is great wellness news. Motivation is essential to success, and we appear well motivated to address life-threatening and otherwise unsatisfactory aspects of our day-to-day behavior.

Unfortunately, most of these change efforts fail to achieve their goals. And most people are trying to make these difficult changes without sufficient support from housemates, family, friends, coworkers and neighbors. Wellness change stories unfold every day and touch all of us. As a result, you've probably heard stories similar to the following.

- Two days of resolve toward weight loss and now a pint of Ben & Jerry's ice cream. After eating the ice cream, Carmen felt that all hope was lost. She wanted the fat to disappear, but just couldn't keep herself on track.

- Jim knew that his wife, Linda, was going to be angry. This was the third day this week he had stopped by the bar after work. He had promised Linda he'd quit drinking. Alcohol really was making his life miserable, but maybe he hadn't hit bottom yet.

- The phone rang and it was another creditor. Jack knew these credit cards were a trap. He thought, "How could I be so stupid? I've been here before. I'm making good money. Why can't I live within my budget?"

- Dr. Larch felt helpless. This was the second child with diabetes she had diagnosed this week, and she couldn't understand why. Pediatricians weren't supposed to treat type 2 diabetes. Weren't these kids supposed to be eating their vegetables and riding their bikes? Dr. Larch hoped that her lifestyle advice to parents would sink in, but she could see that they, too, were out of shape.

- Al kept nodding off. He nearly drove off the road, but was able to pull the big truck off the shoulder and back into the lane. These night hours were murder. The company seminar had warned him of the dangers of sleep deprivation. If only he could get some sleep when off work during the daytime.

- Jane hoped the new health promotion program would meet the needs of her aging workforce and control medical costs. As director of human resources, she understood that employees were counting on getting medical insurance. Still, this year's premium increase would erase all hope for a profit. The CEO and shareholders would not be happy with her report.

- Governor Smith wanted to be known as fiscally conservative, but the rise in state employee insurance, Medicaid costs and Medicare costs were going to cause real pain by forcing cuts in discretionary funding. Still, he believed a tax increase was out of the question. Something had to give. A statewide health promotion program was an option, but Governor Smith was unsure about an effective strategy.

- Rosita was pleased with her husband Juan's medical report. The cardiac rehabilitation was going smoothly. The doctor said that now, after the second heart attack, Juan would really have to eat healthier and get in shape. A heart attack should be a wake-up call, but the last time Juan just hadn't been able to shake his bad habits. This time would be different, or so Rosita hoped.

Each of these stories is both unique and similar. The combination of goals and motivation tend to be unique to the individual. A common thread is that everyone has goals that depend upon lasting and positive behavior change. Eliminating unhealthy habits has both individual and societal benefits. Another common thread is that changing unhealthy habits tends to be difficult. In most cases, effective peer support would dramatically increase the likelihood of success. The best support must be tailored to individual circumstances.

Findings Show the Need for Peer Support

Have you attempted one or more health-related behavior changes during the past year?

If so, how successful were you in achieving your goal or goals?

In 1983, I included these two questions in a study of just over 300 people waiting for their flights at New Jersey's Newark International Airport. Since this preliminary research, I have included these questions (or very similar ones) in more than 100 follow-up studies in a wide range of community and business settings. The answers to these questions have always been very similar. Approximately 80 percent of those completing the anonymous surveys report having attempted at least one behavior change, but fewer than 20 percent report success.

Why do so few succeed? What secret ingredient leads to successful change? It turns out that support is the key. The level and quality of support is highly related to lasting behavior change. Without support at work, at home and in the community, people may attempt change, but are unable to maintain their new desired practices.

The positive role of peer support in behavior change has also been a focus of my research in workplaces. The *Lifegain Health Culture Audit* has been used in several hundred business, health care and education settings to evaluate and plan wellness programs. Survey results show that when most employees attempt behavior change, they experience low to moderate levels of peer support from family, friends, managers and coworkers. When peer support is enhanced via education, support groups and other wellness programs, behavior change success rates rise.

I have found repeatedly that improving peer support is an important tool in creating a corporate culture that supports healthy behavior. Such support influences whether people attempt change and whether they succeed. This is the bottom-line issue for a wellness program. Cost savings and productivity improvements never materialize unless behavior changes.

Clarifying Your Peer Support Role

Wellness-oriented peer support has four qualities that tend to set it apart from other forms of informal and non-paid support.

- Creating a safe and caring relationship for exploring wellness goals. This requires establishing trust and working to keep communications open, positive and guilt-free.

- Asking questions that are useful in planning lifestyle change. Doing more listening than telling. Asking for clarification and reflecting upon what is heard. Those engaged in effective support are more likely to offer more thought-provoking questions than advice.

- Seeking out resources for achieving lifestyle goals. You utilize your contacts and ingenuity to get useful information and to gain needed resources. You may, for example, join your peer in going to the library, surfing the Internet or attending a seminar. You may also join in brainstorming strategies for freeing time for pursuing wellness goals.

- Embracing the learning and growth that come from someone's wellness journey. Your primary concern is avoiding negative judgments and, instead, supporting your peer in taking actions that are heartfelt and truly reflect personal choice.

Your role is different from professional support roles. Unlike those in a professional helping role, you will not be compensated financially for your help. Whereas a counselor or therapist is focused on the deeper psychological causes underlying a behavior, you focus on the practical aspects of health behavior change. You may help your peer find a counselor if deeper and more mysterious problems are identified that need attention.

Although teachers and personal coaches are professionals who guide people with their expertise in a particular area, you are not claiming to be a counseling or health expert. You will ask questions designed to guide your peer toward determining his own best direction, rather than saying what you think is the best direction. You will join together in seeking out useful information from reliable sources.

Drawing Upon the Tradition of Mentoring

The mentor role has its origins in Homer's ancient Greek epic poem *The Odyssey*. Odysseus, the king of Ithaca, had a problem. He was leaving to fight in the Trojan War and needed to find someone who could help his independent-minded son, Telemachus, learn to be a king. Odysseus chose a man named Mentor because he saw that Mentor had special skills. Recognizing that his personal experiences would have limited value, Mentor taught by asking questions. Mentor also saw the value of learning through personal exploration. In this way, Mentor encouraged Telemachus to pursue his natural inclinations. Telemachus was also encouraged to change directions based on what he was learning. Mentor's strategy worked. Telemachus went on to become a helpful son and leader.

As in *The Odyssey*, offering effective peer support does not require direct personal experience with a particular wellness goal. Instead it occurs through the mutual embrace of the learning and growth of a personal wellness journey. Assistance comes primarily in the form of thought-provoking questions rather than advice. You recognize that knowledge unfolds during the process of change. The mentor has faith that her peer can, and most often will, find the best path to his own wellness.

Establishing Trust

Supporting successful health behavior goals usually requires a high level of trust. For many of us this prerequisite can be unsettling. Weren't we taught as children not to trust others? Weren't we taught that change was somehow more valuable if we could claim that we had "done it all by ourselves"? Didn't we learn somewhere that needing others was a sign of personal weakness?

As it turns out, many of these fundamental childhood lessons about distrusting others and not needing them undermine successful behavior change. We need to break out of this dysfunctional attitude about establishing and maintaining trust.

In order to make the concept of trust more manageable, it is helpful to break it down into types of trust. The four Cs of trust are these:

- Contextual Trust

- Communication Trust

- Contractual Trust

- Competence Trust

Contextual Trust

Contextual trust means that our relationship with our peer has a broad basis of familiarity. As we get to know the history and special interests of others, we can begin to appreciate and trust them more. Sometimes this form of trust is established through years of shared life experiences. This could be true of family members or longtime friends. However, all too often, people spend years working and living side by side without really knowing very much about the others' range of experiences. At work, for example, we may know a peer's specific task or job responsibility without knowing anything about her family life, hobbies and personal aspirations.

When thinking about contextual trust, think about the relationship-building skills of successful salespeople. A successful salesperson, sitting down with a customer, does not immediately make sales pitches unless the customer insists. Instead, he opens with a discussion of common personal interests such as hobbies, family responsibilities or sports. He knows that in order to negotiate the best business deal, the two parties must build trust. In a similar way, we should not leap into giving or getting support for health behavior change. First establish a relationship.

By broadening the basis of a relationship, we will feel more comfortable expressing our true feelings and be better able to give and receive constructive feedback. With mutual and broader knowledge of one another, the person receiving the feedback is more likely to experience feedback as having been given in the spirit of helpfulness. In contrast, if all we know about a person is related to one unhealthy behavior, then feedback about that behavior often feels like a criticism of the whole person. When constructive suggestions or probing questions are offered in the context of a broad relationship, it's less likely to feel like a criticism.

Activity for Establishing Contextual Trust

One way to quickly establish contextual trust is to take turns answering "getting to know you" questions. You may want to use the "getting to know you" questions here to help establish trust. Try to share meaningful personal experiences and perspectives without venturing into what should really remain private. Sharing such experiences should be optional – answer only those questions you feel comfortable with.

Tell each other about:

- Places you have lived

- A major change you have made

- Something that would help anyone understand you better

- A childhood experience that has had a lasting effect on you

- A person who has had an important impact on you

- How you chose your present work

- An experience in the last year or two that made a significant impression on you

- An obstacle you've overcome

- A significant personal achievement

- Your hobbies and special interests

Communication Trust

The second "C" of trust, communication trust, refers to the willingness to disclose relevant information. It also refers to using your peer's personal information in a considerate way. When it comes to giving and receiving support for lasting behavior change, accurate and complete information is essential. If you withhold your true feelings, the quality and quantity of support is undermined. In contrast, when communication trust is high, information flows freely. There are five key concepts that build – or detract from – your communication trust:

Confidentiality Agreements

Agreements about privacy help to build trust by outlining how and when personal information may be shared with others. When you are supporting a health behavior goal, there will be times when it could be useful to get input from outside sources. In order to maintain communication trust, you must share information only in a way that has been previously agreed to.

Establish your confidentiality guidelines early. Establish broad guidelines and then check in if unanticipated situations arise. The following guidelines will help you get started. You may want to add a couple of special situations in which personal beliefs, rules or laws dictate the disclosure of information. For example, if you were working with a school bus driver, you might want to state up front that if the conversation indicates that alcohol or other drugs are being used at work, you will find it necessary to contact the employee assistance program or other authorities about the need for assistance. The key is to discuss such limitations on confidentiality in advance. The following guidelines are a good starting place. You may need to add conditions (as the example of helping a school bus driver shows).

Suggested Confidentiality Guidelines

- I recognize that my ability to provide support depends on your confidence and trust in me.

- I recognize that what you tell me is in confidence.

- I will not disclose anything you tell me to anyone without first getting your permission, unless you say that you are planning to physically harm yourself or someone else.

- I will never use the information you give me against you in any way.

The Concept of Need to Know

As we saw in the discussion of contextual trust, it is helpful to get to know each other. However, there are aspects of people's lives that should remain private. Where possible, confine your questioning and probing to relevant information. Encourage your peer to keep conversations focused on wellness goals. Keeping communication purposeful and on topic will help maintain communication trust.

The Obligation to Disclose

Withholding pertinent information or giving false information undermines communication trust. When it comes to behavior change, slips and setbacks can feel embarrassing. Most hunches and feelings are better disclosed and are usually worth exploring even if they are unfounded. Even when information is unflattering, tell the whole truth. Explain yourself fully. Working through hunches and feelings is a good way to establish and maintain trust.

Acknowledging Misunderstandings and Mistakes

A certain amount of trial and error comes with innovation. It is highly likely that at some point you will misinterpret, not communicate well or be misunderstood. It is best to acknowledge such errors, apologize, explain what you have learned, and work toward new understanding. In most situations, there is little value in dwelling on mistakes, but it is important to acknowledge such errors before moving on. This builds trust and enables you to move forward with a minimum of residual baggage.

Attentive Listening

The way we listen enhances or undermines communication trust. We need to know that we are being heard and that our input is being given thoughtful consideration. You can accomplish this by looking at the person speaking, asking for clarification and checking to see if you fully understand what is being said. Bring your focus to what is being said. Try to avoid jumping to conclusions or judging before your peer has an opportunity to fully explain and you have had a chance to digest the information. It's okay to offer your initial reactions, but acknowledge that these are in fact first impressions and not any well-thought-out conclusions. Open your mind to your peer's way of seeing things. Offer your perspective in the spirit of kindness, mutual acceptance and the desire to be truly helpful.

Contractual Trust

Contractual trust, the third "C," is developed when peers come to agreement about how their relationship will function. This doesn't mean that rules are set in stone, but it does mean that the helping relationship will be organized in a way that respects time and other commitments. For example, it is important to establish how often to discuss the peer support goal. You may also need to consider how long you will continue to discuss the goal before you will adjust or end your conversations. Maintaining a schedule, sticking with it and showing up on time are all examples of how to build contractual trust.

Contractual trust includes full disclosure of any benefits or compensation. You should explain why you are offering assistance. The reason can be as straightforward as the desire to help. If you are assisting because you have received similar help in the past, telling that story is likely to build contractual trust. If you are seeking to develop skills for a future career in the helping professions, that should be disclosed. Any form of anticipated compensation should be disclosed.

Competence Trust

The final "C," competence trust, involves respecting people's knowledge, skills, abilities and judgments. To establish this form of trust, you must be clear about your strengths and limitations. For example, you should let your peer know if you have little formal training or experience with an issue that has been raised. An offer of support should not be mistaken for a declaration that you know a great deal about your peer's goals and how they are best achieved. Frank disclosure of experience (or the lack thereof) enhances competence trust.

It is not enough to declare a lack of familiarity, knowledge or skills. You can build trust by accompanying your peer to a library, bookstore or other information source to get needed information. You will build competence trust by actively pursuing useful information. Reading this book is an example of how to build competence trust.

Setting Logistics

When, where and how to meet are important logistical considerations. You will want to come up with a plan that best fits the needs of you both.

Establishing the Format

Ideally, you and your peer will have face-to-face conversations. Such face time provides more complete communication. Facial gestures and body language communicate a lot. Your presence also says much about your high level of personal investment and engagement. Attention span, too, is increased in face-to-face communication. We are less likely to multitask and more likely to listen carefully to someone in our presence. Another benefit of getting together with your peer is physical contact. A handshake and a hug bring us closer together physically and emotionally. They reinforce statements of agreement and our goodwill.

For all these reasons, the two of you should commit to at least some face-to-face conversations. Pick places that are convenient, that allow you to maintain confidentiality, that are relatively free of distracting noise and interruptions, and that are consistent with your wellness goals. Private offices, a booth in an empty restaurant, a picnic table and a walking trail have all served this purpose. To avoid confusion and for increased comfort, try to stick with no more than a couple of places.

Technology brings us a multitude of additional communication formats. E-mail, telephones and Internet chat offer ways to supplement in-person conversations. These are particularly handy when travel is difficult and time is tight. These high-tech and low-touch methods are also helpful in emergencies. There may be times when your peer needs immediate support to get through a particularly challenging day or experience. E-mail and postal mail are nice in that for some people the process of writing helps thinking and commitment processes. Sometimes the emotional distance of writing or using a telephone allows for greater disclosure. You and your peer should discuss possible communication strategies.

Setting Frequency

Peer support is achieved through an ongoing conversation about health behavior change. Momentum is important. Weekly discussions with breaks for holidays, illnesses and family emergencies are one good way to go. Give your discussion times the same priority normally given to work commitments. Follow-up phone calls and e-mail can supplement your weekly discussions on an as-needed basis.

Try not to rush into discussions without first reestablishing your emotional connection. Begin by sharing a little about your life. This will help balance the conversation. You may even add a ritual to the conversation such as a quick sharing of highs and lows for the week. Another example would be to exchange a favorite joke. Time should then be spent on catching up on progress and a review of the past weeks' discussions. Time should also be devoted to discussing a new way to build support.

So, for example, a conversation would begin with a review of the prior week's discussion of health behavior goals and then turn to a discussion of how to identify and work with role models.

One advantage of conversations between peers is that they can continue as long as they are helpful. It is useful, however, to have check-in points so that peer support conversations do not feel like an endless commitment. Two months is a good initial commitment. This will give you an opportunity to discuss most, if not all, of the six different support objectives: helping to set goals, identifying role models, eliminating barriers, locating supportive environments, working through relapse and celebrating success. This time frame will also afford adequate time to make progress on behavior change goals. The two of you should pick a date to discuss progress and the value of continuing to meet. At that time you may also determine that additional conversations can be pursued through other formats, such as phone calls and e-mail.

Peer Support Stories

- John and Jack have great respect for each other as well as a budding friendship. They were introduced through a workplace wellness initiative that paired employees with similar lifestyle goals. Both men wanted to quit smoking. They spent most of their first meeting sharing their personal stories. They quickly agreed to keep their conversations confidential except in cases where someone might be injured. Although it took some hunting, they found a quiet nearby smoke-free café to conduct their Tuesday lunchtime meetings. They also agreed to keep meeting through New Year's Day, as this would be a challenging time for their smoking cessation efforts.

- Alice asked her best friend, Jody, to help her restore balance after a recent divorce. They agreed to keep their conversation in confidence and to take a walk on Wednesday evenings to discuss Alice's goals. Fortunately, they already had a trusting relationship to build upon.

- Jim and Joyce had been married for six years when they decided to make some personal changes. Jim wanted to lose some pounds and Joyce wanted a regular fitness routine. They agreed to hold a special conversation on Thursday nights after their kids were in bed. They also agreed not to discuss their efforts with other family and friends without first getting permission from each other.

- Sabrina finds in-person conversations difficult and prefers the anonymity of online chat. She is working with someone online whom she met in a chat group for breast cancer survivors. After all, she reasoned, I feel a special connection with these people. We've been through a lot and know how to adapt.

- Al and Brendan met at a health spa. Brendan was going through a difficult divorce and was struggling to "get his groove back." Al was exploring his spiritual side and wanted to practice daily meditation. Al felt strongly that Brendan should also meditate. He saw this as the best way to handle feelings about the divorce. Brendan, on the other hand, wanted to pursue a more active social life combined with more physical activity. After their third meeting, Brendan confronted Al about not being open to his wellness goals. Al pushed back and acknowledged that he felt the meditation would do the trick. Brendan told Al that he did not feel the helping relationship was working and asked that they call it quits.

Building the Foundation Checklist

Before turning to the next chapter on help with goal setting, make sure you have built a good peer support foundation. The following checklist will help you determine whether you have covered the core pillars.

☐ We are both clear about the roles and responsibilities.

☐ We see how this support differs from other forms of helping.

☐ We have a plan for how often and where we will meet.

☐ We have identified a good ending date for this round of support.

☐ We have agreed-upon rules for confidentiality, including when we may need to break confidentiality for outside assistance.

Worksheet for Building the Foundation

Questions to Ask	Commentary
1. The Right Person to Help	
Do you see me as a peer?	Find an equal and someone who has a similar frame of reference.
Can we establish a high level of trust?	Look at the potential for contextual, communication, contractual and competence trust.
Do you see me as enthusiastic about your overall wellness goals?	Enthusiasm generates energy and follow-through.
Do I listen well?	Listening is the most important skill in peer support.
Will it be possible to continue to discuss the wellness goals?	Regular meetings help maintain momentum.

Worksheet for Building the Foundation Coninued

Questions to Ask	Commentary
2. Building Trust and Openness	
How will we really get to know each other?	This establishes contextual trust.
Do we have good communication?	Open and honest communication makes the relationship more powerful.
What are the limits of confidentiality?	Decide what rare situations would require breaking confidence (such as a situation in which physical harm or criminal activity is being contemplated).
Do you understand why I am offering support?	Full disclosure of all the reasons for helping builds contractual trust.
What skill and experience, if any, do we have going into this?	Get clear about your skills, or lack thereof, to develop competence trust.
3. Setting Peer Support Logistics	
When and where should we meet?	Decide on a place that is relatively private, convenient and comfortable.
What format will we use to communicate?	Decide about in-person, telephone and e-mail communication and any times when communication should be limited (such as not calling after 7:00 p.m.).
Do I have time for this or am I overcommitted?	A peer support relationship requires thoughtful attention.
What date should we set for completing the first round of support?	Decide on a date so that your conversations don't feel like an open-ended commitment. Then check in to determine if additional support is desirable.

Chapter 2
Setting Goals

At first glance, most wellness goals seem fairly straightforward. In their simplest form, these goals are a description of desired wellness outcomes. For example, your peer might say, "I want to lose some weight," or "I'm going to deal better with the stress in my life."

When you ask for further clarification of the goal, you may find your peer already knows the details of how, when and why the goal will be achieved. If your peer has identified some daily behaviors that will achieve the desired result, you can quickly agree upon benchmarks for success and develop a timeline for achieving those benchmarks.

If wellness goals are already well formed, then your assistance with goal setting will consist of a goals checkup. If, however, the goals are less focused and not fully formed, you will need to turn your attention to supporting your peer in clarifying, refining, integrating and prioritizing the goal or goals.

This chapter explores some of the details that are embedded in goal setting. You will learn how to set goals that are both meaningful and achievable and find strategies for creating these even when there is little clarity about the goal. You will read about how to set goals that are integrated with other priorities.

You will learn about the stages of behavior change that move from initial resistance, through contemplation, preparation, action, maintenance and moving on to other challenges. You will also learn how to get the scientific facts about wellness goals and to separate these facts from wishful thinking, popular fads and marketing schemes. And finally, you will learn how to measure progress.

Embracing the Wellness Journey

Wellness is a process of continual growth. Goals evolve as competing priorities are in flux. Sometimes goals change because people gain new insights. Such changes could be the result of new scientific information or the result of personal experience. Sometimes goals change because the social influences have changed.

Embracing the wellness journey involves resistance to some changes and acceptance of others. Resist making changes that are born out of frustration with behavior change and lowered self-esteem. Embrace changes that reflect a more complete understanding and come from a position of strength and hopefulness. Making such determinations can be extremely difficult; many of our decisions fall into gray areas. You can often come to better goals by clarifying wellness benefits, the social context and how goals fit with other priorities.

Understanding Wellness Benefits

One way to gain clarity on a wellness goal is to determine the benefits that are to be achieved. The following four broad categories offer a way to categorize wellness benefits.

Wellness goals are about:

- **Addressing healing; disease management; and complementary, alternative or integrative medicine.** Sick people want to recover from or manage an illness, and restore vitality. A survivor of a heart attack may be pursuing new diet and fitness goals.

- **Preventing illness and reducing health risks.** A smoker realizes that he is more likely to develop respiratory diseases, cancer and diabetes and has a greater susceptibility to colds, so he decides to quit.

- **Improving quality of life.** A workaholic finds her job overwhelming and unfulfilling, so she drops out of the "rat race" to pursue voluntary simplicity.

- **Attaining peak performance.** An athlete adopts a yoga routine to improve his ability to compete. An artist goes for a morning walk to enhance her creative energy.

With your peer, explore the purposes of achieving the wellness goal or goals. Which of the wellness benefits above are being engaged? Clarifying the primary motivations for change will also guide the type of information that will be useful in planning the change. A goal of regular exercise takes on very different characteristics if it is being used to address heart disease. The advice of a cardiac rehabilitation center is very different from the advice of a triathlon coach. It's best to get information that matches the wellness motivation even if the journey may later evolve into other wellness themes.

Understanding Social Context

Wellness goals are often heavily influenced by others. What is the wellness goal about?

- **Pleasing others.** A son tries to lose weight because his mother is concerned about his health and his ability to attract a woman.

- **Fitting in or being more desirable.** A smoker attempts to quit so she can find a job in a smoke-free company.

- **Caring and being responsible.** A father seeks to cut his risk of a heart attack so that he will live long enough to see his children grow up.

As can be seen in these examples, social motives can be complicated in that they are not under our direct control, and they may be mixed with shame, guilt, fear of rejection and the desire to rescue others. It is tempting to discount the importance of these motives and to recommend that people "get over" or move beyond such influences. But social forces, although complicated, are real and have consequences. They must be factored into any wellness goal.

To be responsible, we must take the needs of others into consideration, but we must also be responsible about living our lives in accordance with our own needs and passions. For example, a goal for stress management must fit with employment considerations. We can't just quit a stressful job without upsetting our economic wellness as well as the welfare of those who count on our paycheck. Clarify how wellness goals affect others.

Integrating Priorities

Wellness goals often address a number of behaviors that overlap in such a way that one goal spills over into other goals. For example, someone wanting to lose weight may find herself achieving this goal as a result of pursuing other goals, including increasing physical activity, reducing job stress, sleeping better and eating healthier foods.

For wellness goals to be fully integrated, they must be organized and prioritized. A better understanding of the breadth and scope of personal priorities will enhance the overall result by identifying possible synergies and by taking potentially competing concerns into consideration.

The following *Wellness Lifestyle Inventory* can be completed by your peer to help determine needs and priorities. It covers a broad range of possible goals within the areas of physical, social, economic and emotional wellness.

Wellness Lifestyle Inventory

Instructions: Most people can identify several wellness goals. This inventory helps you identify some strengths and opportunities for improvement. For each question, you must consider two issues. First, determine whether or not this wellness quality is already in place. Check the boxes for these strengths. Then, decide whether or not you would like to change this aspect of your life. In the second column, check the boxes associated with areas you would like to change.

EMOTIONAL WELLNESS	Achievement	Satisfaction
Rate your achievement and personal satisfaction with your current wellness.	**I already do this**	**I would like to change this**
Start your day rested and with a good attitude.	☐	☐
Rarely feel "blue."	☐	☐
Achieve a balance between work, rest and play.	☐	☐
Balance work and family/household responsibilities.	☐	☐
Rarely feel stress (less than a few times a week).	☐	☐
Take time during most days for prayer, meditation or reflection.	☐	☐
Feel your life is important.	☐	☐
Be in control of your own behavior.	☐	☐
Feel that you are basically a good person.	☐	☐
Feel good about how your body looks.	☐	☐
Use personal mistakes as opportunities to learn and grow.	☐	☐
Laugh regularly.	☐	☐
Find ways to make everyday or routine tasks interesting or satisfying.	☐	☐

EMOTIONAL WELLNESS CONTINUED	Achievement	Satisfaction
Rate your achievement and personal satisfaction with your current wellness.	**I already do this**	**I would like to change this**
Find times to kick back and relax.	☐	☐
Regularly do things that make you happy.	☐	☐
Celebrate personal accomplishments.	☐	☐
Approach life with honesty.	☐	☐
Explore your talents and interests.	☐	☐
Be open to new ideas and experiences.	☐	☐
Follow through on working toward your goals and dreams.	☐	☐
Be in touch with your inner feelings and motivations.	☐	☐
Develop your own sense of spirituality and meaning in your life.	☐	☐
Find ways to make a contribution to the world.	☐	☐
PHYSICAL WELLNESS	Achievement	Satisfaction
Rate your achievement and personal satisfaction with your current wellness.	**I already do this**	**I would like to change this**
Keep your body flexible through regular stretching.	☐	☐
Keep your muscles in tone through lifting weights or some sort of resistance workout.	☐	☐
Enjoy at least two forms of physical activity (such as biking, walking or swimming).	☐	☐
Keep your heart fit by taking part in 30 minutes or more of physical activity most days of the week.	☐	☐

PHYSICAL WELLNESS CONTINUED	Achievement	Satisfaction
Rate your achievement and personal satisfaction with your current wellness.	**I already do this**	**I would like to change this**
Not smoke.	☐	☐
Avoid smoky places.	☐	☐
Organize your home and/or work to avoid injury (including such matters as lighting, lifting, and safety gear).	☐	☐
Wear a seat belt at all times when riding in a car.	☐	☐
Never ride in a car that is driven by someone (including yourself) who has been drinking or is driving recklessly.	☐	☐
For men: consume fewer than 12 alcoholic drinks per week and fewer than 4 drinks on any single occasion, not exceeding 1 drink per hour.	☐	☐
For women: consume fewer than 9 alcoholic drinks per week and fewer than 3 drinks on any single occasion, not exceeding 1 drink per hour.	☐	☐
Avoid activities that place you at high risk for AIDS (including unprotected sex with multiple partners and sharing needles).	☐	☐
Avoid nonprescription "recreational" drugs.	☐	☐
Eat foods that are low in fat.	☐	☐
Eat foods that are high in fiber.	☐	☐
Consume little, if any, caffeine.	☐	☐
Avoid eating refined sugar.	☐	☐
Find ways to prepare and enjoy meals consisting mainly of fruits, vegetables, nuts, whole grains and beans.	☐	☐
Be within 10 pounds of your ideal weight.	☐	☐

PHYSICAL WELLNESS CONTINUED	Achievement	Satisfaction
Rate your achievement and personal satisfaction with your current wellness.	**I already do this**	**I would like to change this**
Brush your teeth at least twice daily.	☐	☐
Floss your teeth daily.	☐	☐
Visit your dentist at least once a year for treatment or a checkup.	☐	☐
Undergo recommended health screenings and physicals.	☐	☐
Have at least one health professional with whom you feel comfortable discussing medical problems.	☐	☐
Look up needed medical recommendations.	☐	☐
Be a careful consumer of medical resources by getting second opinions where appropriate, following through on treatment plans and asking about costs.	☐	☐
ECONOMIC WELLNESS	Achievement	Satisfaction
Rate your achievement and personal satisfaction with your current wellness.	**I already do this**	**I would like to change this**
Sharpen your employment skills through continuing education, reading and discussing your work with others.	☐	☐
Ask for fair compensation for the work you do.	☐	☐
Speak up to stop mistreatment of yourself or coworkers.	☐	☐
Join with others in the workplace in eliminating unsafe products and consumer fraud.	☐	☐
Have a detailed personal financial plan that will achieve your short- and long-term goals.	☐	☐

ECONOMIC WELLNESS CONTINUED	Achievement	Satisfaction
Rate your achievement and personal satisfaction with your current wellness.	**I already do this**	**I would like to change this**
Organize your spending practices so that you live within your means.	☐	☐
Be in agreement about money matters with your spouse or domestic partner.	☐	☐
Comparison shop for the best combination of product, customer service and price.	☐	☐
Avoid materialism (that is, buying because of advertising, sales pressure or just to have what others have).	☐	☐
Save environmental resources and money by fixing and maintaining your possessions, recycling and using less energy.	☐	☐
Pay your credit card bills in full.	☐	☐
Pay your rent or mortgage, utilities, taxes and car payments on time.	☐	☐
Save and invest at least 5 percent of your monthly income for retirement, education or a rainy day.	☐	☐
Have enough financial reserves (not including retirement savings) to last at least 6 months without employment.	☐	☐
Have enough investments or life insurance available in the event of your death to meet the living expenses and tuition of your children until they become adults.	☐	☐
Protect your investments through diversification and by funding your individual retirement account or pension plan.	☐	☐

ECONOMIC WELLNESS CONTINUED	Achievement	Satisfaction
Rate your achievement and personal satisfaction with your current wellness.	I already do this	I would like to change this
Be sure you are getting a reasonable rate of return for the investment risks you are taking.	☐	☐
Have a close friend or family member who would come through for you if you had financial problems.	☐	☐
Be able to help friends and family members with financial problems.	☐	☐
Choose investments that reflect your personal values (avoiding investments in companies whose work harms the environment, for example).	☐	☐
Make purchases that reflect your personal values.	☐	☐
Make contributions to causes and charities that you believe in.	☐	☐
SOCIAL WELLNESS	Achievement	Satisfaction
Rate your achievement and personal satisfaction with your current wellness.	I already do this	I would like to change this
Develop, renew and maintain friendships.	☐	☐
Socialize with friends on a regular basis.	☐	☐
Have at least 2 close or intimate relationships.	☐	☐
Experience the love and affection you need.	☐	☐
Feel close to your family.	☐	☐
Introduce yourself and greet people you encounter.	☐	☐
Regularly get together with others to play games, enjoy friendly competitions, go to the movies or attend community or cultural events.	☐	☐

SOCIAL WELLNESS CONTINUED	Achievement	Satisfaction
Rate your achievement and personal satisfaction with your current wellness.	**I already do this**	**I would like to change this**
Value diversity (appreciating variety in backgrounds and beliefs).	☐	☐
See other people as basically good until proven otherwise.	☐	☐
Respond in others' time of need.	☐	☐
Be a good listener.	☐	☐
Acknowledge your mistakes.	☐	☐
Resolve conflict in positive ways.	☐	☐
Cheer others on.	☐	☐
Share credit for success.	☐	☐
Celebrate the accomplishments of others.	☐	☐
Be honest.	☐	☐
Offer constructive feedback to others in a nonjudgmental way.	☐	☐
Feel comfortable in social situations.	☐	☐
Feel comfortable taking a leadership role.	☐	☐
Team up well on tasks or projects.	☐	☐
Join a support group when faced with continuing (chronic) physical or emotional problems.	☐	☐

Interpreting Wellness Lifestyle Inventory Results

There is no good or bad score for the *Wellness Lifestyle Inventory*. In fact, there is no score at all. Wellness is more about making conscious choices and working toward achieving full potential than it is about meeting a universal standard. *The Wellness Lifestyle Inventory* is designed to raise consciousness about the wide breadth of the wellness philosophy. The following recommendations are for possible follow-up discussions.

- **Review strengths.** Acknowledging those aspects of wellness that are already in place is a good place to start. Explore these positive qualities with your peer. How can they be used to address any remaining opportunities for improvement? Explore how lifestyle strengths were developed. See if you can learn from past successes. Build upon these strengths when approaching issues that still need attention. Wellness strengths are important because they indicate your peer's past success and are the building blocks for his future progress.

- **Review those areas that need attention.** It's okay if your peer's answer indicates she does not practice a healthy behavior and yet is satisfied with the way things stand. It's probably better to look at the areas where there is a desire to change. Try not to impose an opinion, but ask questions to get clarification about her understanding of these areas.

- **Examine any goals not covered in the** *Wellness Lifestyle Inventory.* Determine whether all interests were adequately covered and discuss any gaps or variations that better reflect your peer's personal interests.

- **Explore possible connections between goals.** Wellness is an integrative process that engages mind, body and spirit. By examining possible links among wellness goals, you may come up with new practices that address many goals simultaneously. For example, a daily yoga practice could address stress, flexibility and core body strength. A daily jog or walk could help address weight loss, cardiovascular health and emotional health. Many healthy behaviors, when pursued with friends, can also address social wellness goals. Go over the list of desired behavior changes with your peer and look for ways that any of these could simultaneously achieve a number of positive wellness goals. These changes could be given a higher priority.

- **Examine personal passion, motivation and enthusiasm for the goals.** Wellness goals need to be important enough to inspire continued commitment. Enthusiasm and drive make changes easier to maintain and more enjoyable. The best goals are not always the easiest.

Clarifying Goals

It is likely that your peer has several goals in mind. The following questions help clarify and prioritize these goals.

- **If there is more than one goal, what are the top priorities?** Have a conversation about current wellness goals, including how much change should be taken on now, and whether some goals should be addressed later. Everyone has limits. A change must be important enough to maintain interest and engagement. Goals must be big enough to be challenging but not so big that they feel overwhelming.

- **Do you both have the necessary information to set good goals?** It is important to separate facts from fiction. Try to find information that you have confidence in. Is the information supported by adequate research? Does the source have a reputation for accuracy, or is the information part of a sales pitch? Has the information held up over time and with repeated investigation? Is the information appropriate in terms matching up with your peer's age, sex and other characteristics? You and your peer may need to investigate reputable Web sites, go to a library or consult health experts to get additional input about the appropriate behavioral goals and how they should be achieved.

- **Do you have good ways to measure progress? Ideally, you will be able to regularly assess goal achievement.** Measurement should have a behavioral component. For example, the goal might be to walk three miles most days of the week. Additional measures of progress should also be explored. For example, with a fitness goal, a given resting heart rate may also be a measure of success. Another example would be to be able to talk comfortably while maintaining a certain pace.

Working the Change Process

The focus of lifestyle change efforts evolves over time. A goal of staying on track with a newly established behavior change program has a different focus than does an initial goal of "trying on a desired behavior for size." I've adapted James Prochaska and Carlo DiClemente's six-stage model to create a useful behavior change map.

Share this road map with your peer. Use it to determine the most likely current stage of change. If it is difficult to determine the stage of change, use the series of questions that follow this table to narrow down the alternatives.

The Process of Behavior Change

	Stage of Change	Appropriate Change Goal
1.	**Developing Commitment:** Your peer is not truly convinced about the importance of the lifestyle goal. Your peer may be just exploring the general possibility of taking on a particular goal. For example, someone might have told him such a goal is worthwhile.	If you find yourselves in the "exploratory phase," then the goal is to get more information about the value of such a change.
2.	**Contemplation:** Your peer would like to change and thinks she will attempt change in the next six months.	Your peer should set a date for making the change. Engaging in conversation about the possibilities can often help solidify your thinking.
3.	**Preparation:** Your peer is planning to take action in the immediate future (usually within the next month) and is determining the best strategy to carry out the change.	Together, develop the plan for how the change will be carried out. Your peer should let others know about his intention to change.
4.	**Action:** Your peer is engaged in making changes.	Help your peer adjust to the new lifestyle and manage unexpected emotional and physical reactions.

The Process of Behavior Change (continued)

5.	**Maintenance:** Your peer is working to integrate the behavior change into her normal day-to-day life.	Continue to pay attention to the behavior and work through any relapse. The central focus for your peer is to get comfortable with the new behavior and have it become fully integrated into other aspects of life. Your peer can also mentor someone with similar goals. Teaching tends to reinforce positive changes.
6.	**Moving On:** Your peer has maintained the change for a year or more, and has not been tempted by the old behavior.	Help your peer set new health-enhancing goals. Move on from support systems that are focused exclusively on the prior lifestyle goal. It is no longer useful for your peer to look at himself as one step from relapse. It's time to move on to other wellness interests.

If it is not clear which stage of change applies best, the following questions can narrow down the possibilities.

Questions for Determining the Stage of Change

	Questions to Ask	Likely Stage of Change
1.	Have you begun to adopt the new practice(s) that move(s) you toward your goal?	If yes, skip to question 4. If no, answer questions 2 and 3.
2.	Do you believe that changing this behavior is important to your personal health and well-being?	If the answer is no, you are likely to be in the **Developing Commitment Stage**.
3.	When do you plan to start changing your behavior?	If you express a general interest in changing with no particular timetable, you are in the **Contemplation Stage**. If you have set a date to begin your behavior change, you are in the **Preparation Stage**.
4.	How long have you been practicing your new chosen behavior?	If you have begun the new behavior and have maintained the practice for less than six months, you are in the **Action Stage**. If you have practiced the new behavior for six months or more, you are either in the **Maintenance Stage** or in the **Moving On Stage**.
5.	Have you been tempted to practice the old unhealthy behavior in the past year?	If you are no longer tempted by the old behavior, you are likely to be in the **Moving On Stage**.

The six stages of change provide a useful road map for behavior goals. Use the stages to mark progress and then celebrate success. If things get off track, use the stages to see where the change effort has settled. The road map also keeps conversations meaningful by narrowing the focus. For example, a conversation about how to get started that is appropriate in the preparation stage would not be as useful for a peer in the maintenance stage. In the maintenance stage, the focus would more likely be on issues such as how she can manage a relapse or avoid high-risk situations.

Peer Support Stories

- Greg's mother has Alzheimer's disease. Greg has read numerous books on the subject and has received information from the Alzheimer's Prevention Foundation. He recently read a New York Times article that said getting exercise and taking aspirin regularly could prevent the disease. Greg now feels as if he is an Alzheimer's expert, but he has yet to make a behavior change. Greg has talked about his goals with his officemate, Bill. They have determined that Greg is ready to set a date to begin his exercise program. He is ready to add a 20-minute walk to his daily routine. They are satisfied that they have a plan that would address Greg's prevention goal.

- Jill wants to cut 10 minutes off her next marathon time and qualify for the Boston Marathon. She asked for support from her husband, Bob. They hunted for advice in a stack of recent Runner's World magazines and also reviewed a book by several top women marathoners. Jill and Bob used these sources to come up with a list of possible changes. They settled on incorporating some shorter speed workouts into Jill's routine and upping the amount of daily stretching. They decided to wait until after the New Year's holiday to begin these changes.

- Stan is approaching retirement. He asked his friend Steve about his own recent retirement and Steve suggested that they help one another make the transition. Stan and Steve completed the *Wellness Lifestyle Inventory*. Both men came up with some goals for each of its wellness dimensions. When setting priorities, Stan decided to focus on social wellness. He was particularly concerned that he would feel lonely without his work buddies. Steve identified economic wellness as his first priority. He hadn't anticipated that his post-work life would be so expensive, and he hoped he could find new activities that were less costly.

- Alice's heart attack was a wake-up call for her entire family. The hospital offered nutrition counseling, and Alice attended cardiac rehabilitation for the next month. Alice was getting good guidance from her medical team and was making progress toward a full recovery. Alice's oldest daughter, Jen, was particularly concerned that Alice take all the right medications. Alice was happy to have Jen's support, and they both attended a meeting with the nurse to go over each drug. Alice's husband, Jared, wanted to help Alice lose weight and get an exercise routine going. After some discussions, Jared realized that Alice wasn't interested in exercise, but was excited about healthier eating. They looked over a number of weight-loss programs and settled on Weight Watchers because it had a good track record and seemed to match Alice's overall philosophy.

Goal-Setting Checklist

Before turning to the next chapter on identifying role models, summarize your goal-setting findings. The following checklist will help you determine whether you have covered the key ideas.

☐ We examined the underlying thrust of our wellness goals. We have determined whether the goals are directed at (1) managing an illness, (2) lowering the risk of future health problems, (3) improving quality of life, or (4) achieving peak performance.

☐ We looked at the social context for the wellness goal and how relationships may be influencing decisions.

☐ We examined the overall wellness picture to reveal a range of wellness goals. We determined how some goals could be accomplished together. We prioritized the goals or determined which goal should happen first, second, third, and so on.

☐ We investigated the facts pertaining to the wellness goals. We identified the best sources of information available for setting specific, measurable, short-term and long-term goals. Our goals make the best use of available science and research. The approaches we are taking have shown their worth in situations similar to ours.

☐ We discussed the six stages of the behavior change process. We have benchmarks for moving along the stages toward our wellness goal(s).

Worksheet for Setting Goals

Questions to Ask	Commentary
1. Embracing the Wellness Journey	
What are the main purposes for achieving the goal?	Wellness goals are often associated with addressing an existing illness, preventing future illness, improving overall quality of life, achieving peak performance or some combination of these.
What is the social context for achieving the goal?	Sometimes wellness goals are set to please others, to fit in, to be more desirable, to be caring of others and to be more responsible.
What are the behavior change goals?	Identify behavior change goals associated with emotional, physical, economic and social wellness.
What are current behavioral strengths?	Identify strengths associated with emotional, physical, economic and social wellness.
Are there ways that current strengths can be applied to new wellness goals?	Strengths encourage forward movement.
Are there some actions that will address two or more behavior change priorities?	Many wellness activities, such as yoga, stopping smoking and physical activity, have a number of payoffs.
What wellness goals is the changer passionate about?	It takes energy and passion to achieve many goals.

Worksheet for Setting Goals Continued

Questions to Ask	Commentary
2. Clarifying Goals	
If there is more than one goal, what are the top priorities?	Review the findings of the previous questions to identify priorities.
What information is needed to set a good goal?	Wellness goals such as diet and exercise often lead to recommendations for short- and long-term goals as well as strategies for achieving those goals.
How will progress be measured?	It is easier to see progress when goals are clear, specific and measurable. Such feedback keeps goals on track.
3. Working the Change Process	
What is the current stage of change?	Knowing the stage facilitates focusing on the tasks that are most meaningful.
What will indicate forward movement to another stage of change?	The stages form mini-goals and a road map for seeing progress as the behavior change unfolds.

Chapter 3
Identifying Role Models

Role models offer a window into a successful future. Why wait to see the benefits of change when others have already achieved the same or similar goals? Why not look at what has worked? Why not avoid some of the common mistakes and pitfalls? Why not get encouragement from someone who has walked in the same shoes? Visualizing success through a role model can speed progress.

You may find it a relief to know that you are not expected to be your peer's role model. It is unlikely and unnecessary for you to have achieved the same or similar wellness goals. You can work with your peer to seek out one or more role models. You can help select the best role models. You can help take full advantage of a role model's experiences.

Exchanging Success Stories

A good way to begin the conversation about finding a good role model is to relate the task to your own experiences. Most of us have experiences that make us role models for some sort of behavior change. It is likely that your stories include successes that will inspire. Think about goals you have achieved and obstacles you have had to overcome. Your peer is also likely to have achieved some successes. Exchange stories and recollections of times in your lives when you have achieved wellness goals.

Ask:

- What was your wellness goal?

- What were the reasons you made the change?

- What strategies worked?

- What challenges did you overcome?

- How did other people help?

These are the same questions that might be asked of a future role model. You will be looking for someone with the capacity to answer such questions as they relate specifically to your peer's wellness goal.

Finding Role Models

Begin the search for people who have achieved your peer's wellness goal. Don't be discouraged if finding good role models requires some digging. These are private stories and it is frequently considered bragging to openly discuss successes. Although a couple of candidates could be enough, try to brainstorm and track down a larger list of candidates before settling upon your final choices. The following strategies are good ways to start.

- Look among family, coworkers, friends and acquaintances. Think about the various groups you belong to. Has anyone mentioned a similar wellness goal? These people are often open to a face-to-face discussion as well as follow-up support.

- Ask family, coworkers and friends if they know someone who has achieved a similar wellness goal. You may be pleasantly surprised about their contacts. A friend of a friend is often open to being of assistance.

- Find a local course or support group that focuses on your goal. The teacher or recent course graduates make knowledgeable role models. Many people continue to attend support group meetings well after they have achieved their goals. These people are often enthusiastic, willing to help and knowledgeable.

- A company wellness program coordinator or employee assistance program counselor may suggest some candidates who are willing to be contacted. Some helping professionals keep an active list of wellness role models.

- Chat rooms and discussion groups are now common on the Web. These conversations often focus on wellness goals. You can find them by searching www.Google.com or www.Groups.Yahoo.com. The participants in these discussions can be helpful role models.

- Personal stories, sometimes known as blogs, are also common online. An Internet search on a wellness goal may turn up one or more blogs created by potential role models.

- Associations have programs dedicated to wellness goals. Many of these groups are organized to address a particular disease. For example, the American Cancer Society offers smoking cessation programs. The local chapters and the national organization will help identify role model candidates, suggest Web resources, offer support groups and provide literature with success stories.

- Self-help books and DVDs feature wellness success stories. Libraries, bookstores, DVD rental stores and online shops like Amazon.com are good sources. Many books in the medical and self-help section include personal testimonials. The authors frequently relate their own experiences to illustrate key concepts. DVDs are now available on most wellness topics and feature eligible role models telling their stories in a compelling and entertaining format. The main disadvantage of these role models is that they tend to be inaccessible. It is unlikely that you will be able to establish an ongoing conversation with the creator of the content. Some sources, however, will reference Web sites that support conversations with the author or with other readers.

Sizing Up Role Models

An effective role model provides inspiration, insight, encouragement and an appreciation of the many benefits of successful change. The following table describes key qualities to seek out and those to avoid in a role model.

Role Model Qualities

Qualities of an Effective Role Model	Qualities of an Ineffective Role Model
Has achieved similar goals under similar circumstances.	Has achieved a goal that differs in important ways. For example, an obese person's effort to lose 60 pounds is substantially different from the effort of an overweight person to trim 5 pounds.
Recognizes that great benefits were realized through successful lifestyle change.	Views his own change efforts as more trouble than they were worth.
Is willing to share her story, including the difficult parts.	Shares nothing about personal experience beyond that it was successful.
Is willing to take time to tell his full story and to establish trust.	Is not able or willing to share his experience and build trust.
Sees change as a process.	Expects quick fixes.
Is not quick to criticize or to judge.	Immediately makes character judgments.
Believes it is important to get support from others and shares how other people played a role in her success.	Thinks change is best achieved without the support or involvement of others.
Acknowledges that change can be a challenge.	Says that change is easy.
Gives others permission to create their own path to success.	Recognizes only one way to success: "my way."

Use this table of role model qualities to help your peer narrow down a list of possible role models to the best candidates. The table may also be helpful in conversations with a new role model. Sharing some of the qualities listed in the table will help clarify the type of support your peer is seeking. The qualities may also be useful later on. Use the list to see whether your peer has gotten the full benefit of his or her relationship with a role model. For example, you may want to probe deeper for the challenges your role model experienced in achieving his goal.

Connecting with a Role Model

You may want to help think through the best way to approach a role model candidate. Asking someone to be a role model can be a tricky proposition. The term *role model* sometimes implies a level of perfection, and many people don't see themselves in this way. A good approach is to explain your peer's wellness goal and to ask a role model candidate if she has achieved something similar. Follow-up questions could flesh out the role model's experience. At the end of the initial conversation, ask if it would be all right to ask follow-up questions as his efforts progress.

Questions for a Role Model

Have a set of questions ready before meeting with a potential role model. This will provide the most useful information and help keep the conversation flowing. The following questions are a good place to begin:

- What did you accomplish?

- What strategies did you use?

- How did you track your progress?

- What were some of the benefits of making the changes?

- What was particularly difficult, and how did you overcome those challenges?

- What help did you get from others?

- Who inspired you or served as your role model?

- What sources of good information did you find?

- Can my peer check in with you after she begins to make changes?

Whenever possible, you and your peer should try to meet face-to-face with a role model. The in-person experience increases the level of communication, allows for personal warmth and enhances believability. Set aside adequate time so the conversation will not be rushed. Forty-five minutes to an hour usually works best.

Peer Support Stories

- At age 51, Rafael had a stroke. He had really been struggling to get on track both mentally and with his rehab program. His wife, Jana, asked a counselor for names of people who'd recovered from strokes. Rafael called a couple of the people on the list, focusing on the men, as he felt he could relate best to guys. The people he called were happy to share their experiences, but they turned out to be much older and well past retirement. Rafael felt that he should continue his search until he could find someone more like himself. They called the counselor for more names. Jana also purchased a book about stroke that included a number of success stories by younger men.

- Joanne is struggling with credit card debt. Her friend Jock wanted to help. Jock had been fortunate enough to avoid credit problems himself and suggested that they look on the Internet for some leads. Jock identified some bloggers who have turned their debt problems around. Joanne is now exchanging e-mail with one of these bloggers. Joanne and Jock decided to attend a seminar on debt problems. They asked the speaker to share success stories. They also asked to be put in touch with successful past participants.

- Steve is getting ready for the 160-kilometer Canadian Ski Marathon between Montreal and Ottawa, Canada. He knows that this will be a big athletic endeavor, so he contacted a good friend, Morgan. His friend had completed ski marathons in the past and offered to provide support. They discussed role modeling. Morgan was glad to share his experience. He also knew a couple of other race veterans and was willing to introduce Steve by hosting a dinner party for them all. At the party, each was encouraged to share fun stories as well as their advice for completing the race. After the party, Steve developed a training schedule. He then asked several of his new friends to review it.

- Ingrid had become concerned about global warming and wanted to change her life so that it would have less negative impact on the environment. She and her husband, Johannes, decided to work together on this goal. When it came to the point of selecting role models, they decided to go to a meeting of activists. A number of helpful books were mentioned, and a couple of the people talked about their own lifestyle changes. Ingrid and Johannes stayed on after the meeting to mingle and exchanged phone numbers with other participants who were likely role models.

Identifying Role Models Checklist

Role models can be of immense inspiration. Role models can offer a beacon, a light at the end of the tunnel, as your peer embarks on a lifestyle change. This means that it's well worth looking beyond immediate friends and family to find the best possible people to fill this role. The following checklist will help you and your peer determine whether you have addressed the potential for working with role models.

☐ We brainstormed sources of role model candidates and determined who will follow up and get contact information.

☐ We discussed role model qualities to get a clear picture of the desired characteristics.

☐ We contacted candidates and began the conversation with them.

☐ We followed up with role models with in-person meetings and progress reports.

Worksheet for Identifying Role Models

Questions to Ask	Commentary
1. Hearing Success Stories	
What are our past behavior change successes?	Sharing success stories builds confidence. It also identifies skills and resources needed to achieve lasting and positive wellness goals.
2. Sizing-up Role Models	
What qualities are you looking for in an ideal role model?	Review the list of qualities of an effective role model and visualize the qualities desired.
What are the selection criteria for prioritizing the list of potential role models?	The criteria may help eliminate some candidates and help determine the most likely candidates.
3. Finding Role Models	
Who are the potential role model candidates?	Identify as many highly qualified and willing individuals as possible.
4. Connecting with Role Models	
What is the plan for contacting potential role models?	Be sure to approach candidates in a friendly way that invites their assistance.
What questions will be asked of the role model?	Organize the interview in such a way that the role models will have an opportunity to share their stories and make useful suggestions.
What will be done to make it possible to pursue follow-up conversations?	Questions and tasks change throughout the behavior change process. Leave the door open for additional input from role models.

Chapter 4
Eliminating Barriers to Change

One of the greatest wellness stories of all time took place on Robin Island just off the coast of Capetown, South Africa. This was the site of a political prison that held Nelson Mandela and other South African leaders for several decades. The prisoners were held in small cells and allowed few privileges. Mandela and the other prisoners recognized that they would need their health if they were to survive and continue their work to end apartheid, so they committed themselves to doing everything within their power to sustain their mental and physical fitness. They exercised in their cramped cells and tried to eat as well as they could. They formed an underground school to sharpen their thinking and to sustain their mental health and well-being.

By their final release in 1990, the prisoners' discipline and creativity were so inspirational that even their once-cruel prison guards had been moved to feel admiration and friendship for their charges.

Their story illustrates what can be done to pursue wellness even under the most oppressive conditions. Fortunately, few of us will ever endure the hardships experienced by Mandela and his fellow prisoners. Most of us experience barriers to wellness that are more of an inconvenience than a true hardship. However, the psychological and physical barriers we experience are *real*.

We often find that we lack the time, equipment and other resources needed to achieve wellness goals. We often find it difficult to justify our wellness activities. And many of us lack the discipline and focus to stick with a plan of action. Your peer undoubtedly has some barriers in the way. To adequately address those barriers, your peer needs your help. You can help find ways over and around barriers to behavior change.

Determining Resource Needs

Successful behavior change frequently requires resources such as time, equipment and the cooperation of others. The following table can stimulate a discussion of the resources typically needed for such an effort.

Resources for Behavior Change

Resource Needs	Discussion
Time	Time is an important ingredient of success. Estimate how much time your peer might need to achieve the wellness goal. For example, if physical activity is the goal, how much time will be spent exercising? Another aspect of time is making the new behavior a regular or routine part of the day. Help your peer find a time when the needed energy levels and equipment are available, and also a time when other commitments will not compete.

Resources for Behavior Change (continued)

Resource Needs	Discussion
Backing	We all juggle our responsibilities and commitments with others. Ideally, coworkers, supervisors, housemates and family will accommodate any shifts in responsibility needed to support your peer's wellness goals. Determine who should be consulted and how to approach them. Determine how responsibilities such as childcare will be covered. If such accommodation is not available, how can these barriers be overcome or worked around?
Equipment	Wellness activities require the right tools. For example, yoga routines benefit from having loose-fitting clothes, a yoga mat and a quiet space with a comfortable temperature. In a similar way, a good garden plot and access to a health-oriented grocery store is important when your peer's goal is to achieve a healthy diet. Determine any equipment that will be needed and how it will be found.
Expertise	Behavior change frequently requires know-how. It will be much easier for your peer to stick with a behavior that he is good at and feels confident about. Formal training, mentoring and self-study can build knowledge, skill and confidence levels. Together, determine the best way to secure the information, practice and skills your peer needs for success.
Focus	Mental health and a positive attitude are important factors in sustaining behavior change. For example, sleep is essential to a healthy attention span and to thinking processes. Anxiety can undermine your peer's focus. Mood also plays a role in achieving wellness goals. Fortunately, many goals, such as exercise and healthy eating, enhance psychological well-being. Determine how any unmet emotional and psychological needs may pose barriers. Make a plan for addressing those needs.

Conducting a Strength Review

Our strengths, not our weaknesses, help us move forward. Barriers can feel overwhelming when we lose track of our strengths. You can help your peer regain forward momentum by conducting a strength review. Review resource needs and ask your peer the following questions.

- **What resources are already available for achieving your goal?** Think about strengths in terms of time, backing, equipment, expertise and focus. Come up with a comprehensive list.

- **How can strengths be applied toward acquiring needed resources?** For example, your peer may have enthusiastic friends (a strength) willing to care for her children while she goes for a daily run.

Breaking Down Barriers

If requests don't work, some obstacles to wellness must be confronted head-on. If social pressures and a lack of resources are standing in the way of wellness, then it is not only appropriate, but also just, to demand that those barriers change. A society is in trouble when someone must be a hero or a martyr to do what's right.

Many support systems for wellness behavior are unfunded and under-resourced. So, for example, if there are too few bike lanes or paths, a peer interested in biking must join with others to demand that such wellness resources be built. If your peer cannot get healthy food at the grocery store, strategies need to be developed to make such foods available. You can work with your peer to demand change. Here's how:

- **Discuss why wellness is a human right.** All people deserve good health and an opportunity to achieve their potential. People should be encouraged to pursue wellness goals, not discouraged. For example, the lack of whole-food restaurants or supermarkets and affordable fitness facilities undercuts wellness. Working long hours or forgoing vacations, which is often seen as necessary in order to "get ahead" or "succeed," also undermines wellness. Explore conditions that undermine growth, especially those related to your peer's goal. Discuss the role of society and social institutions in fostering wellness. Consider whether appropriate requests can be made of the workplace or community. Although changes may not be made as quickly as you would like, you will be paving the way for others who follow you.

- **Develop strategies for working with "gatekeepers," such as a supervisor, coworker or housemate.** Asking for support frequently requires a game plan. For example, a work supervisor is more likely to extend the lunch hour to accommodate fitness if (1) the request is made respectfully, (2) the work still gets done, and (3) the supervisor understands the relationship between health and productivity. With your peer, take turns role-playing such gatekeeper conversations.

- **Discuss what can be done to break down wellness barriers.** Work rules and conditions, government service, laws and the activities of community groups can all support wellness. There is some truth to the saying "the squeaky wheel gets the grease." Ask for needed change. Join with others in advocating for needed organizational and community change.

Coping with Barriers

Behavior change is greatly facilitated when conditions are favorable. But, as was the case for the Robin Island inmates, wellness can be achieved even in the face of adversity. The following coping strategies may help your peer move through any apparent barriers. Advise your peer to:

- **Join with others.** You do not have to do this alone. As we will see in the chapter on locating supportive environments, support groups offer their members tremendous psychological strength and hope and encouragement.

- **Consult role models.** These people have likely experienced adversity and devised good coping strategies. Ask for their ideas and encouragement. See Chapter 3 for more on role models.

- **Change your focus.** A barrier does not negate the benefits of other available resources. Focus on what you want, your strengths and resources, and what can be accomplished. Make it a practice to review strengths and celebrate progress. Positive thoughts make struggle less taxing.

- **Be kind in other aspects of life.** Cut back on other responsibilities. Increase the number of pleasurable activities in your day. Allow for renewal activities such as sleep, exercise and socializing with supportive friends.

- **Use any barriers to mobilize determination.** Barriers, especially when they are unkind, unjust or arbitrary, can spawn outrage and resistance. Take a stand and resist. Don't let injustice and thoughtlessness win.

Peer Support Stories

- Angelo dreams of spending quality time with his wife and young daughter. His officemate, Larry, is working with Angelo to come up with a plan. The primary barriers are an unpredictable work schedule and Angelo's inability to communicate well with his boss (who is truly difficult to communicate with). Larry and Angelo have talked about Angelo's current strengths. Angelo will try to parlay his record-breaking sales year into some time off and a fixed work schedule. He has practiced this conversation with Larry. Larry has reminded Angelo to treat his boss with respect, but to remain firm about his needs.

- Jackie lives in rural Nebraska and manages her daily walk through November, but finds that the winter months are too dark and cold. She's also concerned about getting injured on the icy roads. Her friend Linda is also trying to come up with a way to get through the winter with some kind of exercise program. They are planning on creating a community fitness room at the volunteer fire station.

- Art has arthritis. The pain keeps him from sleeping. His best friend, Jim, is encouraging Art to expand his pain research to include sleep issues. They have talked about napping and about developing an evening routine that will promote good sleep. The nap requires a work break. Art would also need to get a couch for his office. With Jim playing the role of Art's boss, Art and Jim have rehearsed the conversation with Art's boss. Art is pleasantly surprised when his boss reverses his initial decision and agrees to let him take a nap in a conference room. Art notices that his conversation with Jim bolstered his confidence and enabled him to stick with his requests.

- Jan is training for the Lake Placid, New York, Ironman Triathlon, but local traffic makes bike workouts scary. She talked with her friend Chris about her fears. They decided to attend a meeting of the local bike and pedestrian coalition. Since then, Jan has become an advocate for bike lanes. She's written a letter to the editor of the local paper, called the transportation department and brought her concerns to the town planner. She's been promised a bike lane by next year. It's too late for the Ironman training, but Jan is thrilled about her progress in creating a safer community.

Eliminating Barriers Checklist

Barriers can make wellness goals much more challenging to achieve. Addressing barriers requires creativity and good problem-solving skills. Your peer is much more likely to come up with good strategies when the two of you approach resource needs together. The following checklist will help organize your efforts.

☐ We have a clear picture of the resources (time, backing, equipment, expertise and focus) that are needed to achieve wellness goals, and we know of any gaps in resources.

☐ We have reviewed existing resource strengths and how these may be applied to address barriers to change.

☐ We have requested or demanded needed resources.

☐ Where needed, we have engaged the support of gatekeepers such as supervisors, family members and housemates.

☐ Where needed, we have brought down barriers by effectively advocating for change.

☐ We have developed coping strategies for moving forward despite remaining barriers.

Worksheet for Eliminating Barriers to Change

Questions to Ask	Commentary
1. Determining Needs	
What time would help?	Although wellness goals for eliminating negative behavior may free up time, many positive practices, such as physical activity, require time for the new behavior. Ideally, this would be a predictable and regular time that allows for a routine.
What backing or permission would help?	Some goals require that your peer get a release of responsibilities from other tasks such as work or childcare. Permission and cooperation can enhance what will be accomplished.
What equipment would help?	Some goals are best achieved with particular tools, clothes and other equipment.
What expertise would help?	Proper instructions and training make behavior change easier for your peer.

Worksheet for Eliminating Barriers (continued)

Questions to Ask	Commentary
What mental health and attitude issues need to be addressed?	Lack of sleep, psychiatric conditions, anxiety and other mental factors can interfere with change. In contrast, a positive attitude and overall mental health make it more likely that your peer's goals can be maintained.
2. Conducting a Strength Review	
What resources are already available	Take stock of existing resources, as such resources form a base upon which to work.
How can available resources be applied toward getting needed resources?	The people and places that already serve as resources are likely to offer clues about filling remaining gaps in your peer's resources.
3. Breaking Down Barriers	
What is the justification for asking for resources to achieve our wellness goal?	Confidence that the goal is a good one and that it is worthy of needed resources is important to making the case for more resources.

Worksheet for Eliminating Barriers (continued)

Questions to Ask	Commentary
Who will need to cooperate and how shall they be approached?	A strategy should be developed for asking for resources from gatekeepers such as supervisors and family members.
What will be done to tear down barriers?	Sometimes it is necessary to petition for changes in rules, lack of resources and other barriers. Such advocacy can be done solo or by joining with others.
4. Coping with Barriers	
What coping strategies will be used where resources are unavailable and barriers remain?	It is unlikely that change will occur under perfect conditions. Help your peer recognize the barriers and develop workarounds or coping strategies.

Chapter 5
Locating Supportive Environments

What comes to mind when you think of a supportive environment? Perhaps you visualize a tropical paradise or a gathering of smiling friends. A supportive environment does include special occasions and interesting places, but for our purposes right now, we're looking for something far less exotic. We're focusing on supportive daily environmental influences, like the people and the places in your peer's daily routine.

The house, the workplace, the neighborhood and the grocery store are just some of the settings that influence behavior. In a similar way, housemates, spouses, friends, children, coworkers, teammates, club members and neighbors form our immediate social – and hopefully supportive – circles.

Helping your peer find and create physical, emotional and social environments that support his wellness goals is an important peer support strategy. In this chapter I will share how you can bring environmental influences into focus, and how to modify these influences so that they better support your peer's desired wellness behavior. I will draw upon the perspectives of anthropologists, architects and city planners, who are all experts in understanding or creating environments.

First Encounters with Wellness and Positive Support

I first heard the word *wellness* at Frost Valley, the YMCA's largest summer camp, located in the Catskill Mountains of New York State. It was 1978 and I was looking for a job during my high school summer vacation. My father, Robert Allen, Ph.D., had been invited to help teach camp counselors about wellness and suggested that I take a summer job at the camp.

Don Ardell, Ph.D., Bill Hettler, M.D., and John Travis, M.D. (an editor of this book), joined my dad in explaining the wellness concept and how we were to promote wellness among our young summer campers. These guys said that wellness was about good social relationships, managing stress, exercising and eating nutritious foods. We were told that a wellness lifestyle would increase the likelihood of a long and illness-free life. After a week of training, the counselors were enthusiastic about the new wellness initiative.

Everything seemed perfect until the kids started arriving. Their camp trunks were packed with what appeared to be a lifetime supply of junk food and candy. Furthermore, many of the kids had been shipped off to camp because their parents had given up on them and each other. Broken families and psychological problems were commonplace. Wellness didn't look like it was going to come naturally to our campers. They were not thrilled when we described the new camp menu and philosophy.

At our first counselor meeting, we talked about our dilemma. Most counselors complained about the inadequacy of our training. Some questioned whether wellness was such a great idea for our camp. It was clear to many of us that success would be achieved only through addressing peer cultures. Wellness would have to become the new and fun way to do things. We would need to change support systems so that they would promote wellness.

It took some doing, but I'm pleased to report that Frost Valley YMCA was largely successful. We introduced new health-oriented cooking ideas at "the Incredible Edible House" – a converted maple sugaring shack that now made nutritious alternative treats for the campers. We also developed a wellness manual with more than 100 activities designed to introduce various wellness concepts. We incorporated environmental education – a camp strength – into the overall wellness initiative. We revamped chapel services so that kids and counselors could talk about sources of meaning and purpose in their lives. We introduced yoga postures at our morning camp-wide gathering at the flagpole. We helped one another get the most out of our camp experience and the wellness philosophy. Although we did not call it such, our friendships were based on peer support. Our goal was to create a supportive camp environment for pursuing personal wellness.

Finding and Creating Supportive Physical Environments

When an architect plans a house, each room is designed to support its function. The kitchen has a stove, refrigerator, sink, cabinets and countertops. In a similar way, a behavior is easier to achieve with a supportive physical environment. For example, if healthy eating is the goal, access to nutritious and tasty foods is crucial. Grocery stores, restaurants and vending machines should feature foods consistent with your peer's goals.

Focus on helping your peer find supportive places, limiting exposure to unsupportive environments and changing those aspects of environments that work against wellness.

Think about where a new behavior is to happen. Is it:

- Safe?

- Convenient?

- Well-maintained?

- A pleasant temperature?

- Appropriately equipped?

- Affordable?

- Comfortable?

Keep an eye out for unsupportive factors – the opposite of these. Some factors rank higher than others. For example, although Equinox Health Club in New York City meets all but one or two of these criteria, I do not use it because it is beyond my budget and the club near my mother's apartment doesn't have a lap pool.

What can be done to make the physical environment more supportive of wellness goals? Having assessed the physical environment, you and your peer can plan how to change recreational, work and living spaces so that they are more supportive. Consider finding new places. For example, early spring and late fall in Vermont are not conducive to outdoor exercise. A lucky few travel out of state, but many migrate to health clubs and indoor skating rinks. We Vermont residents also set up treadmills and exercise bikes in our homes. The following questions are useful for pursuing supportive physical environments.

- What places support your wellness goals, and how can you spend more time in these places?

- What places are unsupportive, and how can they be changed or avoided?

- How can you find or create new supportive places?

Mobilizing Wellness Buddies

Many people find it easier and more enjoyable to do things with a companion. A wellness buddy is someone who has the same or a very similar wellness goal. It is like a buddy system for child safety at a pool. Both children swim and keep an eye out for each other. A wellness buddy may also be engaged in peer support conversations, but this is not a requirement of a wellness buddy. You can help your peer find one or more wellness buddies.

The power of the wellness buddy approach has worked wonders in my own life. Two days a week, I get together with a couple of friends at 6 a.m. to jog. On Sunday mornings, I do my "long run" with a running club. During these jogs, we talk about current events, our lives and our exercise goals. These times with my wellness buddies are among my best. They keep me energized even though I'm not usually an early riser. My wellness buddies make my fitness routine truly enjoyable. We are in this together.

Consider the following questions when helping your peer establish wellness buddy relationships.

- **Do your peer's wellness goals lend themselves to partnering with another person?** Think creatively about this. Even activities that are generally done alone, such as financial planning or managing an illness, could be done more easily with another person who is pursing similar goals. Such people could be wellness buddies.

- **Who would make the best wellness buddies?**
  Existing social networks often offer good choices for
  wellness buddies. So if your peer is trying to manage weight, she could partner with her housemates.
  Frequent contact and a shared refrigerator enhance
  the benefit. In addition to existing social networks,
  wellness buddies can be found in a support group,
  at a wellness seminar or on the Internet. Use the
  same approaches recommended in the "Identifying
  Role Models" chapter.

- **What are barriers to finding wellness buddies?** In
  American culture there is a myth that the things we
  do by ourselves are somehow more enduring than
  and superior to what we do with others. This has
  been a particularly strong message to men. Let your
  peer know he needs to reach out to others even if it
  stretches him some. Once the ice is broken, people
  usually find that the wellness-buddy approach is far
  superior to the go-it-alone approach.

- **What is the ideal schedule for connecting with
  wellness buddies?** This depends on the wellness
  goal. If the goal involves a routine, buddies can do
  that routine together. Weekly contact helps keeps
  the energy flowing. I joined Weight Watchers with
  my wife and neighbors. We attended weekly meetings together and then went out for sushi afterward
  to celebrate our progress.

Finding and Creating Supportive Cultural Environments

How would anthropologists rate someone's chances of achieving a wellness goal? They would look at the influence of tools, buildings and social networks. They would look to see if wellness behaviors are rewarded. They might also examine rites of passage, rituals and symbols – do they detract from or enhance wellness? So, if eating a cake is way people typically celebrate, they might suspect that losing weight will be difficult. Just like an anthropologist, you and your peer can examine cultural environments to plan how to avoid unsupportive environments in favor of supportive cultural forces.

Some unhealthy aspects of our current cultures are hard to overlook. Such is the case with obvious excesses of a caffeine-drinking culture. American culture's epidemic of overeating is another example of a readily apparent health problem. When addressing cultural support, you and your peer will want to look for the readily apparent markers of the culture and more subtle and less obvious influences. Work with three powerful, but too often overlooked, cultural dimensions: cultural climate, cultural norms and cultural policies and procedures, which I refer to as touch points.

Fostering a Supportive Cultural Climate

When people don't get along, it is difficult to focus on personal growth. In a hostile environment, people are angry, frustrated and uncooperative. In the United States, airports have come to symbolize such settings. The buzz is predominantly negative and filled with suspicion. High security, overbooked flights and disgruntled airline employees keep people on edge. Other common examples of hostile or highly stressful environments are companies undergoing downsizing and families going through a divorce. Help your peer toward either resolving such conflict or finding ways to avoid the daily grind of unpleasantness.

A good climate takes different forms in households, workplaces and neighborhoods. Personal change is much easier to pursue in a friendly and cohesive social environment. In a marriage this might be referred to as the honeymoon phase. On a worksite it's called great teamwork. A strong sense of community, a shared vision and a positive outlook are dimensions of a supportive climate. These factors enhance individual and organizational growth. A sense of community provides for trust and openness. A shared vision enables people to be inspired by a common direction. A positive outlook makes it possible to use individual and collective strengths in meeting challenges. Finding or creating a healthy climate is a useful lifestyle change skill for both you and your peer.

Your peer can examine the climate with the *Cultural Climate Test*. The questions examine the three climatic dimensions.

Cultural Climate Test

Instructions: Focus on one social group or setting at a time. You can repeat the test for the important social groups in your life such as your household, work group, family and community organization. Rate your level of agreement with the following statements on the 5-point scale: (5) strongly agree, (4) agree, (3) undecided/don't know, (2) disagree, and (1) strongly disagree.

	Sense of Community
5 4 3 2 1	I know the people in my group really well.
5 4 3 2 1	I feel as if I belong here.
5 4 3 2 1	Members would support or care for me in a time of need.
5 4 3 2 1	I trust these people.
5 4 3 2 1	I feel comfortable saying what's on my mind.
	Shared Vision
5 4 3 2 1	We share common values.
5 4 3 2 1	I am able to explain the mission of my group.
5 4 3 2 1	I recognize how my own day-to-day activities contribute to the group's mission.
5 4 3 2 1	My group's conduct is consistent with its stated purpose and values.
5 4 3 2 1	My group has a clear and consistent direction.
5 4 3 2 1	Overall, I find my efforts with the group inspiring.

Cultural Climate Test (continued)	
	Positive Outlook
5 4 3 2 1	I am proud of the contribution my group is making.
5 4 3 2 1	My contribution to the group is recognized.
5 4 3 2 1	Achievements are celebrated.
5 4 3 2 1	We have a sense of humor about challenges we face.
5 4 3 2 1	We have a "can do" attitude.
5 4 3 2 1	Conflicts are resolved in positive ways.
5 4 3 2 1	Difficult assignments are treated as special challenges and opportunities, rather than problems.
5 4 3 2 1	I feel optimistic about the future of my group.

Scoring the Cultural Climate Test

The maximum score on the test is 95. Few groups achieve this ideal, but you and your peer can use the answers to identify ways to improve the climate. If most individual item scores are 3 or lower, your peer should consider limiting exposure to this group.

With the help of the *Cultural Climate Test*, your peer can quickly understand the climate concept and how to assess the various social environments in her life such as her household, workplace, church or neighborhood. Then the two of you can use these questions to develop a strategy.

- **Do some of your peer's social environments lack a supportive cultural climate?** If "yes," decide whether that is likely to change, what can done to turn it around and whether it is best to disengage. Focus on ways to minimize contact with hostile or toxic environments your peer can't change.

- **Do some of your peer's environments provide a supportive cultural climate?** If "yes," how can your peer more fully benefit from them, and how can people in this setting become involved in supporting your peer's wellness goals?

- **How will your peer find settings with good climates?** Search for positive environments and ask an insider questions like whether people get along and if morale is good. Use the *Cultural Climate Test* questions as a guide in observing whether a sense of community, a shared vision and a positive outlook are evident. Some environments are difficult to read. In my neighborhood, for example, the annual summer picnic, beach cleanup and neighborhood meeting would be the only times to get a full read on the neighborhood's social climate. Until you had been at the picnic, you would not fully appreciate the positive spirit of the neighborhood.

Working with Cultural Norms

In a supportive culture, desired behavior is the normal practice. People would be surprised if you behaved any other way. In a fitness-oriented household culture, for example, housemates would talk about their daily exercise plans and share responsibilities so that everyone got time for physical activity. Housemates would share tips about hiking, biking and other interests. Fitness achievements would be celebrated.

Cultural norms are usually so embedded in the social fabric that we don't notice their influence. One quick test for a norm is to see if your peer gets "pushback" from a group. If the behavior is against the norm, people are likely to get concerned, and your peer is likely to hear statements like, "Around here, we don't do it that way." If it is a norm, the behavior will either meet with approval or go unnoticed. After all, it is "the way we do things around here."

Assess the norms in your peer's social environments to determine the level of cultural support for wellness goals. The following questions may help:

- Which social settings have norms that are for, neutral, or against your peer's wellness goal?

- How can your peer minimize exposure to groups with unsupportive norms?

- Which groups, if any, already have strong norms that support your peer's wellness goal?

- How can new groups with supportive norms be found or created?

- How can exposure to groups with supportive norms be maximized?

Working with Cultural Touch Points

A culture touches its members in subtle and not-so-subtle ways. If norms represent what is expected of people in a culture, touch points are the social mechanisms that establish and reinforce those expectations. Touch points, like reward systems, reinforce the behavior. Touch points are often embedded in formal and informal policies and procedures. For example, there may be a formal orientation program for a new employee offered by the human resources department and there is likely to be an informal orientation by coworkers that occurs on the job or over lunch.

In a family culture, most of the touch points are informal. For example, a family may discuss nutrition while at the grocery store or at the dinner table. This would be the informal communication system that influences goals for healthy eating. The following questions examine such cultural influences.

Examining Cultural Touch Points

Instructions: Keep your peer's behavior change goal in mind when discussing answers to the following questions. The questions examine how a group, family or organization hinders or promotes the desired wellness behavior.

Touch Points	Positive Influences	Negative Influences
Rewards and Recognition	Is the wellness behavior rewarded and praised?	Is undesired or unhealthy behavior rewarded and praised?
Modeling	Do leaders model the wellness behavior?	Do leaders model unhealthy behavior?
Confrontation	Is unhealthy behavior effectively discouraged or confronted?	Is the wellness behavior discouraged or ridiculed?
Relationships	Do people tend to form friendships while practicing the desired wellness behavior?	Do people form friendships around unhealthy practices?
Training	Do people get the training and skills needed to excel at the wellness behavior?	Are people taught skills that would make them more comfortable with unhealthy practices?

Examining Cultural Touch Points (continued)		
Touch Points	**Positive Influences**	**Negative Influences**
Orientation	Does the orientation (formal and informal) of new people give a first impression that the wellness behavior is the norm?	Are new people given the impression that unhealthy practices are acceptable?
Communication	Are people given feedback about how they are doing with the wellness behavior?	Would people be unlikely to have their wellness behavior noticed or assessed? Are such practices unmeasured and unreported?
Rites, Symbols and Rituals	Do celebrations, holidays and special events reflect support for the wellness behavior?	Do celebrations tend to feature unhealthy behavior?
Resource Commitment	Does the use of time, space or money show that the wellness behavior is important?	Are there inadequate resources available for the wellness behavior?

Many touch points work in unison to influence behavior. However, it is likely that some are giving contradictory messages. For example, a parent may communicate that he values healthy eating yet may be a poor role model when it comes to healthy eating. Other touch points may be sending no signals. For example, there may be no discussion of healthy eating in a family.

It takes power and influence to change touch points. If your peer does not have such authority, it is at least helpful to be aware of these influences and to advocate for needed change. If your peer has power, as is often the case within a family, a group of friends or immediate coworkers, then help your peer work to adjust the touch points so that they better support wellness goals. The following ideas are often useful in thinking about adjusting cultural touch points.

- Many of these influences may have gone unexamined by group or organizational members. When these influences are revealed, members may be open to making changes.

- Efforts to change the influences frequently require decision-making authority or the support of those who have such authority. Try to get the decision makers engaged in addressing the touch points.

- It is not necessary to create an entirely new system or to address all the negative influences. For example, there may already be a system for rewarding positive practices at work. Encourage your peer to see if wellness behaviors can be recognized with this existing program. We are often better off making adjustments in existing influences.

- Start with the influences that will have the biggest impact and are easiest to change. For example, it may be easier for your peer to make changes with her work group or family culture.

Each of your peer's cultural settings contributes to determining the overall influence on her wellness goals. Each has its own touch points. For example, the workplace culture may offer predominantly positive influences, whereas the household culture may undermine wellness goals. Ideally, the overall impact will be positive. However, it is likely that one or more settings will not fully support the wellness goal. As with negative norms and dysfunctional cultural climates, your peer will find it helpful to reduce contact with environments that have touch points that work against a wellness goal. Another tactic would be to increase contact with settings that are more likely to have a positive influence.

Peer Support Stories

- Joanne is helping her husband, Sam, get back on his feet after being laid off. Sam feels cut off and isolated. They discussed some possible wellness buddies. Sam was reluctant to connect with his former coworkers because they constantly complained about their old employer. Joanne suggested that Sam go down to the local office of employment and training. Sam called ahead and signed up for a seminar on interviewing. During the break, Sam met a couple of guys he liked. They decided to meet once a week over lunch and support each other in their job search.

- Angela was trying to cut back on her drinking, but her fights with Ramon really made it hard. Her best friend, Deb, offered to provide peer support. Deb asked about the cultural climate at home. Most conversations between Angela and Ramon quickly turned into shouting matches. Angela and Deb talked about the household climate and realized that something would have to change. Angela convinced Ramon to go with her to a counselor, and as they progressed, Angela also made progress with her drinking problem.

- Laura and her officemate, Derek, were obsessed with work and knew that this level of obsession was unhealthy. They decided to help each other. Both immediately noticed that the norm was to work 60 or more hours a week. Many coworkers bragged about working though the weekend. Laura and Derek called a team meeting to discuss job burnout and the possibility of creating a healthier work culture. There was near-universal agreement that the work culture had gotten out of hand. They discussed policies and procedures with their team. A number of policies were adopted, including keeping track of work hours and setting the weekly individual limit to 50 hours. Laura and Derek were relieved that they would not have to make these changes alone.

- Crystal and Alice were partners. They had been together for 30 years and were both approaching retirement. They listed the environmental qualities they were seeking for their future retirement. They wanted a community that would be open to their lesbian relationship. Ideally, the setting would have norms for an active retirement. They wanted foreign language and yoga classes. Crystal had recently been to San Miguel Allende, Mexico, on vacation. The town was alive with older adults who were exploring their dreams. They decided to visit to see if it would be a good fit.

Locating Supportive Environments Checklist

Before turning to the next chapter on working through relapse, use the following checklist to determine whether you and your peer have addressed important features of the environment.

☐ We have explored the possibility of developing wellness buddy relationships.

☐ We have looked at physical environments and found ways to make them more supportive of wellness goals.

☐ We have assessed the cultural climate and have found ways to limit contact with hostile or otherwise unsupportive environments. We will increase contact with settings with strong senses of community, shared visions and positive outlooks.

☐ We have identified cultural norms that support wellness goals. We have developed a strategy to become immersed in environments where our desired behaviors are "the way we do things around here."

☐ We have looked at cultural touch points embedded in formal and informal policies and procedures. We have found ways to increase desired influences and to lessen undesirable influences.

Locating Supportive Environments Worksheet

Questions to Ask	Commentary
1. Locating Supportive Physical Environments	
What is the ideal place and setup for your new behavior?	Think about a place that is safe, convenient, well-maintained, a desirable temperature, appropriately equipped, affordable and comfortable.
What places support the wellness goal and how can more time be spent in those places?	The right place makes wellness behaviors easier.
What places are unsupportive and how can they be modified or avoided?	It is hard to continue do something if a space is not right.
How can you find or create new supportive places?	New surroundings offer an opportunity to pick places that are specifically chosen for their positive attributes.
2. Mobilizing Wellness Buddies	
Do your wellness goals lend themselves to partnering with another person?	If privacy is not a priority, then almost all wellness goals lend themselves to forming a wellness buddy relationship in which both people take on the same or similar goals together.
Who would make good wellness buddies	Start with existing social networks and housemates and, if necessary, look into support groups, wellness seminars and the Internet.

Supportive Environments Worksheet (continued)

Questions to Ask	Commentary
What are barriers to finding a wellness buddy?	Your peer should reach out to people to discuss wellness goals even if this means stretching the comfort zone. Role-play the conversation to get more comfortable. Most people are open to being asked.
What is the best schedule for connecting with wellness buddies?	Ideally, wellness buddies will do some of their new behavior together, so coordinating such activities is important.
3. Locating Supportive Physical Environments	
What is the ideal place and setup for your new behavior?	Think about a place that is safe, convenient, well-maintained, a desirable temperature, appropriately equipped, affordable and comfortable.
What places support the wellness goal and how can more time be spent in those places?	The right place makes wellness behavior easier.
What places are unsupportive and how can they be modified or avoided?	It is hard to continue to do something if a space is not right.
How can you find or create new supportive places?	New surroundings offer an opportunity to pick places that are specifically chosen for their positive attributes.

Supportive Environments Worksheet (continued)

Questions to Ask	Commentary
3. Locating Supportive Cultural Environments	
What social settings, if any, have a hostile climate?	It will be important to spend less time in settings that lack a sense of community, a shared vision and a positive outlook, as such settings sap energy and are distracting.
What social settings, if any, have cohesive climates?	It will be helpful to increase time in these settings, as they enhance personal functioning and are good sources of social support.
What social settings have cultural norms that fail to support the wellness goal?	If a behavior is against the norm, it will be difficult to maintain. Contact with such settings should be limited.
What social settings have norms that support the wellness goal?	If desired behavior is also the norm, it will be easier to maintain that new behavior. Contact with such settings should be maximized.
What cultural touch points support the wellness goal?	It is helpful to take advantage of touch points that may reward or otherwise endorse desired behavior.
What cultural touch points work against the wellness goal?	Strategies must be developed to reduce or work around these unsupportive influences.

Chapter 6
Working through Relapse

Wellness goals can be a great challenge. They involve changes in daily practices and sustained effort. They often require that we overcome ingrained habits, distractions, or chemical addictions, and that we continue despite deep and long-standing psychological wounds. And, as we saw in the last chapter, we are likely to encounter many physical and social obstacles.

Given this, it is hardly surprising that most people do not achieve wellness goals on their first try. Some goals take many attempts before they are achieved. Your peer must learn how to address the possibility of relapse and how he can move forward beyond the shame and doubt that often accompanies a setback. You can offer support at this important time.

Preventing Relapse

A great deal can be done to avoid relapse. Many of the best strategies have been described in previous chapters. We can avoid relapse by setting meaningful and achievable short- and long-term goals. We can get the facts and base our goals on the best scientific evidence. We can visualize success and learn from the experience of role models. We can lower daily obstacles to change. We can find or create supportive social and physical environments. Together, these peer support strategies create assets that reduce the likelihood of relapse and failure.

Additional relapse-prevention approaches are aimed at avoiding high-risk situations. These questions can help you and your peer identify approaches to staying on track.

- Are there places that should be avoided? An alcoholic beginning recovery should stay away from bars. Identify the equivalent high-risk circumstance for your peer's wellness goal.

- Are there social circumstances that should be avoided? Maybe tensions at family gatherings make progress with overeating or stress management unlikely. Identify the groups and social activities that place your peer at risk.

- Are there times of the day or week that are difficult? For example, being tired often impairs judgment. Slow risers may find early morning a time of higher risk. Help your peer identify the times or days that may be challenging so strategies can be developed for working around the most vulnerable times.

- Are there emotional states that are high-risk? Anger, sadness and fear often throw us off track. Help your peer identify the triggers for such emotions. Strategies for staying on track should be developed for these times.

Checking In

Schedule frequent meetings to discuss progress during the time the new wellness behavior is first being adopted. Lag time is an important factor in working though relapse. It is best to get back on track as soon as possible. So, for example, when I set a goal of cutting back on caffeine, I probably should have gotten some help soon after my first cappuccino. It was not long thereafter that I slipped back into my undesired practice throughout the day. I might have stuck with my goal if I had reexamined my commitment and approach right away with a supportive peer.

Even though relapse is common, it is best not to set an expectation for relapse. A discussion of how to address relapse should begin with the understanding that this is a "just in case" plan. Your hope is that relapse will be avoided and that your peer's progress will be steady.

Addressing a Relapse

Working through the emotional and physiological fall-out of swings in wellness behavior requires great kindness, understanding, creativity and resilience. The following topics make it easier to address the "just in case" of relapse.

Restoring Adult-to-Adult Communication

Feelings of failure tend to make us feel small and guilty – more like a misbehaving child than an adult. Thus, for someone who has experienced relapse, there is a tendency to see others as parents – possibly angry or disappointed parents. This does not make for a good peer support relationship. We cannot be helpful or constructive in this parental role with our peer. No adult finds it satisfying to feel like a child who has misbehaved. To manage these feelings, your peer will most likely avoid other people who treat her like a child.

Effective peer support requires getting back to a conversation between two equals – between two adults. You can bring the relationship back to balance using the following strategies.

You can:

1. Make clear that you are not a judge or a parent and that you see your peer as an adult.

2. Remind your peer that relapse is common. You can offer an example of how you got off track during your own past behavior change attempts.

3. State that your respect does not depend on what your peer decides about continuing his efforts to achieve his wellness goal.

4. State that your immediate goal is to find out what happened, including the facts and the circumstances, and to determine – together – how to proceed.

Interpreting Relapse

Listen for both facts and feelings. Was this a stumble or a true fall? A person thrown from a horse could get right back on the horse, decide to wait for a better horse, or decide that horseback riding is not such a great idea. What scenario fits best? Consider these choices:

- **Maybe this was a stumble and your peer still sees herself as moving forward.** This would be a good interpretation of the experience because it maintains a sense of momentum. Perhaps there are some lessons that the stumble revealed about avoiding future troubles or about managing such incidents.

- **Maybe your peer views all momentum as lost and believes it is necessary to start over.** If this is the case, you should state your enthusiasm for a new beginning. Then you can use the experience to adjust strategy and your support.

- **Maybe your peer wants to wait before starting over.** If this is the case, you can acknowledge the decision and review some of the reasons for making the change with your peer. What would tip the balance toward making another go? What factors would determine when to make another attempt?

- **Maybe your peer has had enough of this goal.** If this is the case, you can acknowledge the decision and review possible alternative plans. What changes in goals or strategy make sense? For example, if your peer is trying to address weight, he may want to change his goal from following a diet to increasing physical activity. You can offer assistance with any new goal.

Getting Out of a Funk

There is little doubt that a setback can be discouraging. Fortunately, Martin Seligman, Ph.D., a founder of the field of positive psychology, has developed a number of strategies for regaining optimism. When your peer encounters a problem, she can choose to interpret that problem as a pessimist would or as an optimist would:

An Optimist's Interpretation	A Pessimist's Interpretation
My troubles are *not permanent*. They will soon go away.	My troubles are here to stay. I will always need to put up with this failing.
My troubles are *not pervasive*. This issue is limited in scope.	My troubles will ruin my entire life and spread over into other previously satisfactory things I have done.
My troubles are *not personal*. They are mostly caused by factors that are not my doing.	My troubles are my fault. I brought them upon myself and no one and nothing else is to blame.

Helping your peer move toward the optimist's position is a useful strategy for raising his spirits after a slip or relapse. Examine the situation to look for reasons the relapse is not permanent, not pervasive and not personal. The strategy only works if your peer believes it is the truth. Look for credible reasons for your peer to take the position of the optimist.

Fortunately, as we have seen throughout *Healthy Habits, Helpful Friends*, there are many external factors that help determine behavior change outcomes. They are at least partially responsible for any relapse.

Unhealthy behaviors don't have to be permanent. The new positive interpretation of the event can lift the cloud of failure and shed new light on the situation.

Peer Support Stories

- Vince is helping his friend Dave break his drug addiction. They discussed the possibility of relapse, and Dave acknowledged that he had been fighting his addiction unsuccessfully for more than 10 years. They discussed those "learning experiences" with an eye toward improving the chances of success. Dave was convinced that making strides in establishing new physical and social surroundings were going to be a big help. Dave was going to make a special effort not to hang out with anyone who had a drug problem. He was also going to avoid alcohol over the holidays and stay away from those places and parties where he knew he would be pressured to drink. Vince and Dave agreed that, no matter what happened, they would remain friends and maintain an adult-to-adult relationship. For the time being, they would check in with each other daily.

- June had set some big goals for diet and exercise after her heart attack. She had befriended another survivor, Arlene, in the cardiac rehabilitation program, and they were using *Healthy Habits, Helpful Friends* together. June had a rough time sticking with her exercise routine. Arlene knew there was something up because June was hesitant to talk about her progress. It was getting awkward, and Arlene decided to clear the air by sharing her hunch. June readily shared her frustrations and the two had a laugh over how June's husband behaved when she put on her workout clothes. They talked more seriously about resetting goals to make them more doable. They also talked about getting June's husband on board.

- Lauren and Clay have a 3-year-old daughter. They were both frustrated at the dropoff in their sex lives. The first thing they agreed about was that it was not easy to balance work and family responsibilities. They were having a hard time coming up with a time when they both had the energy for sex. Juggling new parenting responsibilities seemed like a higher priority. They agreed to be patient and focus initially on getting some fun time together as a couple. To that end, they found a babysitter and declared that Tuesday would be date night. Their wellness goal had changed, but they felt hopeful about their future together.

Working through Relapse Checklist

Before turning to the next chapter on celebrating success, see if you and your peer have planned for possible relapse. The following checklist helps determine whether the two of you have covered the important aspects.

☐ We developed ways to avoid situations that may trigger a relapse.

☐ We set check-in times so that setbacks can be discussed soon after they first appear.

☐ We affirmed our goal of maintaining an equal adult-to-adult relationship regardless of how or whether wellness goals are achieved.

☐ We explored the range of possible setbacks and recognized that we can move forward after a relapse.

☐ We examined whether our helping relationship was still helping.

Working through Relapse Worksheet

Questions to Ask	Commentary
1. Preventing Relapse	
What social situations should be avoided?	Some people and social events are triggers for the old behavior. They raise the risk of relapse and should be avoided.
What places should be avoided?	Some places trigger old and unwanted behavior. They raise the risk of relapse and should be avoided.
What times of the day or week are particularly difficult and what can your peer do to pay special attention during these times?	Coping methods can be used to make it easier to get through those times when your peer finds the old behavior most tempting.
What emotional states are high risk and how can they be avoided?	Sadness, anger, frustration, fatigue, and other feelings can throw us off. Efforts should be made to limit such mental states and to develop coping strategies.
2. Checking In	
How often will we check in, so that any relapse can be discussed early on?	It is important to stay in touch with your peer to offer encouragement and to address relapse issues.

Working through Relapse Worksheet (continued)

Questions to Ask	Commentary
3. Addressing a Relapse	
How will we make sure that we return to adult-to-adult communication?	When a relapse occurs, it is common to feel like a misbehaving child. It is important for your peer to quickly return to feeling like an adult.
What is the result of a relapse in terms of next steps?	Determine if: (1) the goal has been abandoned, (2) a decision has been made to start over, or (3) a temporary stumble has occurred.
How will we regain optimism and get out of a funk?	A relapse can be less draining if it is interpreted as temporary, narrow in its impact, and not entirely your peer's fault.

Chapter 7
Celebrating Success

Too often, successes go unacknowledged. Unheralded success does more than undercut our good cheer. It is a missed opportunity to reinforce desired practices. This is particularly true with wellness goals in American culture, in which daily practices are considered private endeavors and progress sharing is called bragging.

An unintended side effect of the "go it alone" approach is that no one even knows when benchmarks are set, let alone achieved. In the health-care setting, for example, privacy agreements forbid sharing, even when it's good news.

Advocates of the quiet approach go on to praise the value of self-achievement and self-responsibility as if help from others somehow taints successful behavior change and downgrades the achievement. "She did it entirely on her own" becomes a special bragging right. I have come to understand, however, that often, when someone "does it on her own," it is a sad sign of a disconnected society and a strong indication that the changes will be short-lived. We want and need to celebrate together.

Celebrating All Along the Way

One of the best things about peer support is that peers actively seek opportunities to celebrate – and there are many to be found. This goes well beyond the typical approach of celebrating only when the ultimate goal is achieved. Consider the possibilities for celebrating success.

You celebrate when:

• Your peer completes the Wellness Lifestyle Inventory and determines that she already has many great wellness strengths.

• Your peer sets a wellness goal.

• Your peer finds a role model.

• Your peer gets input from the role model. This is also an opportunity to appreciate the role model's input.

• Your peer eliminates one or more barriers to change.

• Your peer finds people and places that will support his wellness goal.

• Your peer develops strategies for limiting contact with unsupportive environments.

• Your peer develops and implements strategies for avoiding relapse.

• Your peer gets back on track after a relapse.

• It is the anniversary of a significant achievement.

In addition to this list, there are times to celebrate that correspond to the stages of behavior change discussed in the *Healthy Habits, Helpful Friends* chapter on goal setting. Each stage has its own transition and marker. These should be celebrated. The following table describes these changes in broad terms.

Transitions Included in Prochaska's Stages of Behavior Change

Transition	Marker
From Developing Commitment to Preparation	Date set for making the change.
From Preparation to Action	Personal changes begun.
From Action to Maintenance	Early adjustment shifts to long-term sustainability.
From Maintenance to Moving On	New lifestyle is completely comfortable – peer is ready to move on to other goals.

Dividing up behavior change by stages offers several opportunities to celebrate. When your peer moves from thinking about change to setting a time to make that change, it is time to celebrate. When she has finished preparing and begins to make the behavior change, celebrate again. Celebrations are also in order when behavior changes have been successful for a short period. When your peer's changes have taken hold several months or a year into the effort, it is once more time to celebrate.

Tuning in with Intrinsic Rewards

Good celebrations often include rewards. Such rewards come in two forms: **intrinsic** and **extrinsic**. An intrinsic reward is a benefit that directly results from behavior change, for example, feeling more energetic after becoming fit. An extrinsic reward is a benefit from another source. The 30-day sobriety chip of Alcoholics Anonymous would be an example of an extrinsic reward.

Most wellness goals result in multiple intrinsic rewards. Someone with a wellness goal of addressing breast cancer might gain an intrinsic reward of being free of cancer signs and symptoms. She might also learn how to manage great personal threats and challenges. The process and achievements may have proven to be a great source of self-discovery and an opportunity to establish new personal priorities. These would all be intrinsic rewards.

Explore the intrinsic rewards likely to result from your peer's efforts and ultimate goal achievement. What are all the intrinsic benefits? Achieving wellness goals lowers the probability of getting sick and reduces recovery time. In addition, many wellness-related behavior changes improve job performance and mood. Your peer's wellness achievements may directly benefit those he loves. Stopping smoking, for example, improves health outcomes for his children.

Some benefits are surprising. Did you know that stopping smoking improves sexual performance? There is a lot of scientific information about the various health consequences associated with unhealthy and healthy behaviors. You and your peer can review this information to uncover some wonderful rewards.

Getting Rewarded by Others

Extrinsic rewards are the way peers, groups and society reinforce wellness. For example, your peer could reward you with praise, a card or some other form of acknowledgment. Similar informal rewards are available from other peers, such as family, friends and housemates. For example, a man who has lowered his cholesterol might comment that one great reward was the look on his wife's face when the results came back.

Organizations and society also have rewards for wellness activities, such as incentives for completing company health risk appraisals. Good health could lead to job promotions, since advancement is often linked to personal productivity and people tend to be absent from work or a lot less productive when they are sick. There are also rewards associated with competitions. I appreciate the T-shirts and medals I get for competing in fitness events.

Sometimes extrinsic rewards are criticized because they are considered a distraction from intrinsic rewards. Other criticisms concern how external rewards are often temporary and not controlled by the person making the change. It does at first appear odd to pay someone for doing something that offers great intrinsic health benefits. However, in most cases it is best to have a powerful mix of intrinsic and extrinsic rewards. For example, stopping smoking is a great accomplishment with direct intrinsic health benefits for those who quit. However, extrinsic rewards, such as lowered health insurance deductibles for nonsmokers, do not undermine the intrinsic rewards. Extrinsic rewards just make the behavior change even more rewarding and are likely to get the attention of those who have yet to pay attention to the intrinsic rewards.

You can help your peer tune in to the intrinsic health and self-esteem rewards *and* make sure that she gets all the external perks, pay and praise available for her achievements.

Refining the Reward Systems

As can be seen with the list of reasons to celebrate and with the variety of intrinsic and extrinsic rewards available, there are many ways to make celebrations meaningful and appropriate. The following questions can assist with tailoring celebrations to best suit your peer's needs.

When you celebrate:

- What are the desired levels of privacy and how will they be maintained? As a general rule, public disclosure and commitment work in favor of successful behavior change. It is a lot harder to give up or go back once your peer has declared his intentions and progress. However, your peer may not want particular people to know about any changes under way. Who should and should not know? How can you celebrate and yet maintain desired confidentiality?

- How can you make rewards compatible with wellness? In American culture, many common rewards are inconsistent with a wellness message. For example, a piece of cake is not an appropriate extrinsic reward for successful weight management. Exotic fruits make a good alternative. A new outfit could be a more fitting reward for your peer. We must often be creative and willing to break with tradition to create a wellness reward system.

- Are there savings that can be applied toward financing a grand prize? When I stopped drinking diet soda and fancy coffees, I put the money into a travel fund.

In the course of a couple of years, these savings made it possible for me to take my grandmother on a cruise to Alaska. See if your peer's achievements offer some savings or another financial benefit. Avoiding illness adds to productivity and reduces costs. Can some or all of this money be redirected toward a fitting reward?

- What are your peer's favorite ways to celebrate? We all have our preferences – our favorite way to relax, our favorite healthy foods, our favorite way to exercise, our favorite places. Rewards should be tailored to personal taste. What is the nicest thing anyone ever said to your peer? Maybe the tone and spirit of that comment can be mirrored in how wellness achievements are celebrated. For example, I particularly found it satisfying when my father talked to me in private about how proud he was of my professional achievements. I favor similar private acknowledgments of current wellness achievements. Some people find monetary rewards most meaningful. If this is the case, see if a family member or your peer's employer would be willing to reward change with cash or a check.

- Are there special celebrants? Perhaps certain esteemed friends, family members or coworkers would offer particularly meaningful rewards to your peer – intrinsic or otherwise. Expressions of delight from a spouse, an "attagirl" from the boss, or praise from parents may carry special weight.

Talk with your peer about some of the rewards that would be meaningful to him. It is sometimes necessary to apply for rewards. The classic example is when we make a wish list for holiday presents. With wellness achievements, for example, it might be necessary to bring your peer's good health and productivity to the attention of a supervisor and alert her about your peer's desire for a promotion. In a similar way, if acknowledgment from your peer's husband would make a good reward, then he would need to know about progress and be keyed in about the hoped-for praise.

Finishing Strong

If you and your peer have organized your efforts in the same sequence as in this book, then you may be reaching a good check-in point for your wellness efforts. Presumably you and your peer have discussed and worked with the six primary peer support strategies of goal setting, identifying role models, eliminating barriers to change, locating supportive environments, working through relapse and, with this chapter, celebrating success.

Take stock of your relationship:

- Spend a few moments in appreciation of your time together, the trust you have maintained, your commitment to success and your ability to adapt.

- Discuss what each of you has learned in terms of peer support and how best to approach behavior change in the future.

- Decide how you will work together in the future. Include in this conversation any new goals that should be considered, time commitments and any other adjustments. For example, you may decide that by a certain date it would be a good time to meet less frequently, or to move to a check-in format with telephone calls and e-mails.

- Find some way to celebrate your relationship. This celebration could take the form of a symbol of your appreciation or a special meal or a shared fun event.

Peer Support Stories

- José and his wife, Rita, are supporting each other to achieve environmental goals for energy conservation. They have adjusted their thermostats and reorganized their work so they can commute two days a week by public transportation. They are tracking their heating bills and travel costs. Half of their savings will go to environmental causes and the rest will be spent on a bike trip across their state.

- Tyler has set a wellness goal of spending more time with his son. His friend and coworker Mark is assisting. Tyler has been thinking about making this change for the past six months and has set New Year's Day for putting his plan into action. Mark offered to take Tyler and his son out to celebrate Tyler's commitment. The three whooped it up at a local college basketball game.

- Ernie and his cousin Paula stopped smoking a year ago on April 5. Another family member, Claire, is supporting their efforts. Claire put together a surprise party for the anniversary. More than 20 family members sang an adaptation of "Puff the Magic Dragon" at the big event.

- Emina has been helping Sarah with her weight. They talked about progress. The conversation turned to some of the rewards she could anticipate. Sarah was looking forward to climbing stairs without losing her breath. Sarah also knew that her weight had become an issue at work, where she was required to do a lot of walking. She worried about what all the walking was doing to her knees. Emina asked if there were any additional rewards that might be fun. Sarah's eyes brightened as she said, "I could buy a new wardrobe."

Celebrating Success Checklist

See whether you and your peer have a good plan for celebrating success. The following checklist helps determine if you have covered the important aspects.

☐ We have identified several times to celebrate, when plans are made and when goals are achieved.

☐ We have compiled a comprehensive list of intrinsic rewards (such as health and well-being benefits) that are likely to occur if we are successful.

☐ We have identified extrinsic rewards (such as pay, bonuses and gifts) that will be available as a result of the wellness effort.

☐ We have discussed strategies for tailoring celebrations and rewards so they are appropriate and meaningful.

☐ We have celebrated our relationship by checking in and by honoring our time together.

Celebrating Success Worksheet

Questions to Ask	Commentary
1. Celebrating All Along the Way	
Have we identified several reasons to celebrate?	Many successes go unacknowledged, which undermines positive energy. It is important to look for the many opportunities to acknowledge your peer's wellness efforts.
What are the markers for the transitions in the stages of behavior change, and how will these transitions be recognized and acknowledged?	The six stages of behavior change offer a road map for focusing your peer's efforts, and moving one stage forward deserves a celebration.
2. Tuning In with Intrinsic Rewards	
What are the health and quality-of-life rewards for your peer when he achieves his wellness goal?	Such benefits include feeling more energetic, increasing personal performance, reducing a health risk, healing and living longer. Some benefits will readily be felt and others may require a review of the scientific literature.
How might your peer's success with the goal benefit others?	Many wellness goals benefit others. This benefit may be important to your peer. For example, when someone quits smoking, it may improve indoor air quality for family members and lessen the likelihood that your peer's children will smoke.

Celebrating Success Worksheet (continued)

Questions to Ask	Commentary
3. Getting Rewarded by Others	
How will your peer's successful behavior change be acknowledged?	Lowered health risk and positive practices sometimes trigger rewards such as lower insurance premiums, financial savings, praise and other forms of extrinsic rewards. It may be necessary for your peer to apply for such payoffs.
4. Refining the Reward System	
What degree of privacy is desired with rewards?	Some people are less comfortable with public acknowledgment, so their rewards need to be low-key.
How will rewards be made compatible with wellness?	Standard rewards may be inconsistent with a wellness message, so it is often necessary to create more healthful strategies.
Will your peer experience financial savings from the behavior change, and can this money be incorporated into a reward?	The savings are easy to see if the old practice cost money, but other savings of time, fewer absences and reduced health care costs can also be factored in.
Are there special celebrants who should be involved with the rewards for achieving wellness goals?	Family members, friends and mentors could add meaning to rewards by being involved with acknowledgment of your peer's change.

Celebrating Success Worksheet (continued)

Questions to Ask	Commentary
5. Finishing Strong	
What has been useful and enjoyable about the peer support relationship?	Reflect on the positive qualities of the relationship, how it evolved, how challenges were overcome and what was accomplished.
How will your relationship be acknowledged?	Celebrate your relationship and how it has enriched both of your lives.

Chapter 8
Bringing On the Wellness Revolution

Congratulations! At this point in *Healthy Habits, Helpful Friends*, you have read about and hopefully experienced the power of effective peer support in bringing about lasting and positive behavior change. You are now ready to explore the broad social implications of the wellness movement and to apply your peer support skills to advancing the wellness cause.

This chapter affords an opportunity to learn about the importance of wellness in society and your role in promoting healthy lifestyles. "Bringing On the Wellness Revolution" explores the potential of wellness to address important societal problems. It also explores the potential for using peer support to bring about needed organizational and societal change. The primary purpose of this chapter is to give you some of the information you may need to advocate for the ideas and skills expressed in this book.

Wellness is truly a revolutionary vision that holds great promise for prevention, healing, peak performance and improved quality of life. Being part of the wellness revolution requires making changes in the way we live. Physical activity, good nutrition, adequate sleep, stress reduction and the avoidance of substance abuse play important roles in wellness. Healthy social connections are another part of the wellness revolution. These connections extend to the state in which we leave the world for future generations.

Peer support weaves together the wellness domains of personal behavior and social connection. By enhancing the quality and quantity of social support, we increase the likelihood of success. Furthermore, efforts to offer effective support enhance human connections. Helping people with behavior change has been primarily the domain of the therapist and wellness professional. I believe that extending this helping role to our peers can bring on a wellness revolution.

Curing the Epidemic

There is an epidemic of destructive health practices in North America and in many other parts of the world. The proportion of Americans who adhere to all four of the most basic lifestyle prescriptions for health – not smoking, maintaining a healthy weight, eating adequate fruits and vegetables, and exercising regularly – is a dismal 3 percent, according to a 2005 study of 150,000 adults. Steven Aldana, author of *The Culprit & the Cure,* tells a tragic story of an America caught in a spiraling epidemic of unnecessary suffering and premature death.

The following facts from *The Culprit & the Cure* show why it is so important that we begin to change our health behaviors.

- Consider some of the recent findings for the United States.

- o 1 out of 4 adults smoke
- o 2 out of 3 adults are overweight or obese
- o 3 out of 4 adults don't get enough exercise
- o 4 out of 5 adults eat an inadequate diet
- Americans are losing ground even among children. Over the past 40 years, the number of American children who are overweight has quadrupled. Physical inactivity is also on the rise. The projections are for widespread diabetes among children.

Research findings regularly report the benefits of a wellness lifestyle. For example, a California study determined that those who exercise regularly, do not smoke, and get adequate sleep have a death rate from cancer and cardiovascular disease that is 70 to 80 percent lower than that of the rest of the nation. The impact of this short list of health practices on life expectancy is staggering. Males with these health practices live an average of 11 years longer and females live an average of seven years longer than average Americans. Research has also found that not only is a person adopting healthy practices more likely to avoid chronic conditions, but her final years are more apt to be healthy ones.

The benefits of a wellness lifestyle are compelling, but the dire consequences of unhealthy behavior are even more so. Once you appreciate the connection between unhealthy practices and poor health, the economic consequences of the epidemic become obvious. Poor health undermines productivity. People can't work as well when they are sick. Poor health requires a lifetime of expensive and otherwise unneeded medical care. To cut the risks of catastrophic illnesses, health professionals are performing surgeries and prescribing drugs to address health issues that would be best treated with behavior changes such as a healthy diet and exercise.

Cleaning the Poisoned Cultural Well

Most epidemics can be traced to a source. The classic public health example is a poisoned well in London. The people in the vicinity of the Broad Street pump were getting sick. John Snow, a London physician, figured this out and removed the pump's handle; the illness vanished.

In the case of unhealthy behavior, cultural environments are the most likely source. The culture is the poisoned well. Smokers learn to smoke through movies, their family and friends. Television and computer games, primary tools for couch potatoes, are social inventions. Bars, parties and alcohol ads have their role in making people susceptible to substance abuse.

Given the many negative influences in North American culture, it is tempting to tell people to go it alone – it's just too hard to get support to do what you want to do. But, just as the residents of London could not do without another source of water, humans require social contact to survive and thrive. Healthy practices can have social roots. Those who exercise regularly, for example, probably learned and were encouraged in developing their fitness skills through a coach, family member or friend. The question is not really whether we will have social contact, but rather whether this contact supports our wellness.

As was pointed out in the chapter on locating supportive environments, we can help each other achieve health behavior goals by finding supportive wellness buddies, changing cultural norms and organizational policies and creating cohesive social climates. With peer support strategies such as these, we can begin to clean the poison from the well of unsupportive cultures at home, at work and in the community. "Locating Supportive Environments" begins a conversation about cultural change. You can further explore this important subject at www.healthyculture.com. The Web site features surveys, training and publications about cultural change.

Connecting

Throughout this book, I have explained how people can help each other achieve wellness goals. Using peer support techniques, you and your peer can make dramatic and lasting behavior changes. Together, you can achieve success rates that would not be possible without support.

If this book has any role in your success, then it was well worth the writing. But the very act of people coming together has a benefit that may far exceed the health benefits and personal satisfaction described here. There is strong evidence that human connection is, in and of itself, as powerful a positive life force as any health behavior change. The very act of reaching out to help someone in constructive ways enhances your own health and the health of your peer. And the connections you are making enhance the well-being of your workplace, your community, your country and the planet.

Promoting Health with Human Interaction

The book *Love & Survival,* by cardiologist Dean Ornish, is a masterful summary of research on the health benefits of human connections. Dr. Ornish cites more than 100 studies that make a compelling case that love, intimacy and human connections prevent illness, heal disease and extend life. The following quote summarizes Dr. Ornish's findings:

- Do you have anyone who really cares for you? Who feels close to you? Who loves you? Who wants to help you? In whom you can confide?

- If the answers are "no," you may have a three to five times higher risk of premature death and disease from all causes – or even higher, according to some studies. These include increased risk of low birth weight and low Apgar scores, heart attack, stroke, infectious disease, many types of cancer, allergies, arthritis, tuberculosis, autoimmune diseases, alcoholism, drug abuse, suicide and so on. A reduction in premature death was found in people who had close relationships. Also people are much more likely to choose life-enhancing behaviors rather than self-destructive ones when they feel loved and cared for.

There is parallel evidence that the health benefits of human connection accrue to those providing support. In one study of more than 700 elderly adults, the more love and support they offered, the more they benefited themselves. Just as with this population of elders, offering peer support has direct health benefits for the person offering support. Such support reinforces your own positive health practices. And it is harder to advocate a healthy behavior for someone else while continuing a contradictory behavior yourself. In addition, as you help others with behavior change, you learn and reinforce skills useful for achieving your own wellness goals. When you help your peers adopt healthier practices, you create a peer culture that is more supportive of your own wellness.

Succeeding at Work

How do you gauge success at work? Your list might include a good salary, a boss who gives you the freedom and support to innovate and do your job well, friendly and mutually supportive coworker relationships, decent work hours, good benefits and job security. Although the quality of your workplace depends on a variety of market forces, government regulations and other external factors, constructive social relationships play an important role in your success as an employee or employer. *In Good Company*, a book published by Harvard Business School Press, describes the role of social relationships in business success. The authors, like many economists, consultants and sociologists, define positive relationships as social capital:

Social capital consists of the stock of active connections among people: the trust, mutual understanding, and shared values and behaviors that bind the members of human networks and communities and make cooperative action possible.

In Good Company reviews many research findings and case studies that link social capital and positive business outcomes. With good social relationships, workers find it easier to voice their concerns and to join with others to have them addressed. Trust and openness make relationships with customers less problematic and legalistic. Good social relationships give people the space, time and constructive feedback needed to innovate. Collaboration and teamwork make it more likely that people will follow through on commitments. In addition, social capital increases morale and job retention. The end result is that good social relationships make work more enjoyable and profitable for all concerned.

In Chapter 5, "Locating Supportive Environments," I focused on a specific aspect of social capital – social climate. We saw how a supportive social climate makes it easier for people to change their behaviors. Your assignment was to help your peer examine the social climate and to limit contact with those environments that lacked a sense of community, a shared vision and a positive outlook. We saw the importance of seeking out and spending more time in groups and settings that have these climatic factors.

But peer support has an impact on social capital that goes beyond boycotting some settings and seeking out others. Peer support for wellness plays a constructive role in generating good work relationships. When it is applied in a work setting, social capital rises. Here's how:

- Peer support for wellness provides employees with a way to help one another and to build mutual trust. Participants learn more about each other – beyond job functions. This broader relationship provides for better communication and trust. The camaraderie associated with taking on big lifestyle challenges carries over into other work functions. Wellness-related peer support is like a rope-climbing course or an adventure retreat, in that personal risk is paired with the enthusiasm and support of coworkers.

- Wellness-related peer support offers an alternative to adversarial relationships and hard times. Too often, economic and other business factors pit people against each other. People in a work group may see themselves as competing for scarce resources. A company may be conducting layoffs or cutting pay and benefits. When wellness-related peer support is offered at the workplace, the "wins" that result can counterbalance the negative and divisive consequences of some business practices.

- Wellness-related peer support connects people who might not otherwise meet. When employees are paired for mutual support, matches can be organized around compatible schedules or similarities in behavior goals. These wellness matchups can mix employees of various job functions, levels of seniority and power. This enhances cross-functional communication, fosters an appreciation of other work groups and helps employees feel connected with the corporate identity.

- A peer support initiative at the workplace puts a human face on business. Some businesses sell themselves short by focusing exclusively on product and profit without seeing the value of their people. In such a climate, an employee is likely to be viewed by shareholders and senior managers as a cost of doing business rather than a human asset. In contrast, where people examine their wellness goals and share them with others, they become unique contributors who are valued in the workplace.

- Wellness-related peer support aligns human and economic interests. This is a major achievement of a healthy corporate culture. Personal goals and work goals are often compatible, and also complementary. As we saw with health behavior and illness, achieving wellness goals provides less costly, more productive and more dependable employees.

Wellness-related peer support enhances social capital in a multitude of ways. However, there are limits to the impact of such support. Peer support does not directly address some of the structural factors that may be undermining social relationships. For example, it may be that organizational leaders are not focused on creating a good work atmosphere, or, as is more likely the case, they do not know how to effectively address their work climate.

If you are passionate about doing more to address social capital at your worksite, you can learn more about the subject by taking the training at www.healthyworkclimate.com. And you can join with a peer to consider how you might engage your leaders in the value of addressing social capital in the workplace.

Bowling Together

Do we have enough opportunities for experiencing kindness and connection? Robert Putnam, author of *Bowling Alone*, conducted an extensive analysis of research on this question and found a recent decline of more than 20 percent in many aspects of social relations. Professor Putnam found that we used to belong to clubs, know our neighbors, engage in community politics, volunteer, eat with family members and host dinner parties. Such social activities have become increasingly rare. The overall trend was summed up in the demise of social bowling throughout America. Whereas we used to bowl in leagues, we now tend to bowl alone.

Professor Putnam looks at the benefits of social relationships in terms of broad societal outcomes. He says that social bonds are the most powerful predictor of life satisfaction. For example, getting married is the equivalent in terms of happiness of quadrupling your income, and attending a club meeting regularly is the equivalent of doubling your income.

In contrast, the loss of social bonds is revealed in lower educational performance and more teen pregnancy, child suicide, low birth weight and prenatal mortality. The quality of social relationships is a strong predictor of crime rates and other measures of neighborhood quality of life. Positive wellness-oriented relationships such as the one you have created by supporting a peer in lifestyle change are a bridge from the negative influences of social groups. For example, this approach would turn around college alcohol abuse and street gang violence.

Professor Putnam calls for new social mechanisms that respond to modern times. He points out that permanent employment is largely a thing of the past. Traditional family relationships are no longer the norm. Suburban sprawl means that people tend to work, shop and live in different areas. With this shift in lifestyle, the likelihood of chance meetings with friends is diminished.

Leisure-time activities have changed, with many technologies such as TV and the Internet offering a substitute for face-to-face interaction. Even architecture is playing a role, as fewer homes are built with front porches.

Wellness-related peer support offers a mechanism for re-building social bonds in modern times. The one-to-one connection can adapt to modern work and living arrangements. A mix of in-person, telephone and e-mail conversations fits today's needs well. Because traditional family roles and work ties have broken down, peer support for wellness offers a new way to build caring relationships and an additional reason to connect with peers. It doesn't rely on traditional family configurations or old-style hierarchical decision-making structures. With peer support we are not managing or manipulating people. This is not a way to get others to do what we think they should do. Instead, we are empowering people to help one another as equals – as peers.

Effective peer support for wellness adds modern "oomph" to social relationships. It offers a format and content for solid helping relationships. Many of us have lost the art of connecting. We have been "bowling alone" for so long that we feel odd spending time with others. We also feel awkward because relationships have been devalued and manipulated. Tupperware parties and network marketing have turned many friendships into a commercial enterprise. Wellness-related peer support reclaims helping for the sake of helping. It is commercial-free. It is a healthy way to "bowl together."

Creating Opportunities for Peer Support

As I stated in the introduction, "A Call to Kindness," a primary purpose of *Healthy Habits, Helpful Friends* is to make peer support less threatening, more effective and more available. The idea of learning to give and receive effective peer support is a new idea that goes beyond the typical self-help approach. The peer support discussed in *Healthy Habits, Helpful Friends* is many notches up from the informal or chance peer support that most of us have experienced. As with any new idea, you will need to reach out and explain to others how this form of peer support works. You should soon have some successful experiences to share. Real-life stories tend to be persuasive. In addition, I recommend that you offer your peers a copy of this book.

I believe that *Healthy Habits, Helpful Friends* can play an important role in enhancing your wellness and the wellness of the people in your life. I also believe that this approach to powerful peer support can help bring about the wellness revolution that is so urgently needed to ensure the well-being of individuals and the planet. Your love and support can be instrumental in making this happen. I count on you to spread the word by sharing your peer support stories.

Please reach out to your peers when you see them struggling with personal change. Lend them your copy of this book and encourage them to get support. Show a peer how to support you when you need it. I also hope that you will recommend *Healthy Habits, Helpful Friends* to people in workplaces, health-care settings and community groups.

Looking to the Future

Keep your peer support skills fresh. Review the book and revisit the many questions and assignments here. You'll be surprised at how your interpretation of these recommendations and your perspectives about effective peer support will evolve over time.

The book draws on many years of research, personal experience and wisdom offered by many health and wellness professionals. The www.wellnessmentor.net Web site includes research reports and online training concerning peer support programs for business and community settings. The Recommended Books section after this chapter features works that may be particularly helpful in reinforcing key peer support ideas and in broadening your perspectives on wellness and helping relationships.

You can learn a great deal from others who are engaged in peer support. To further enhance your skills, consider participating in continuing education opportunities offered at the annual National Wellness Conference (www.nationalwellness.org). I look forward to seeing you there.

Peer Support Stories

- In Michigan, the City of Kalamazoo's wellness council was seeking to increase the capacity of citizens to get involved in supporting each other. The council set up a training initiative that focused on peer support. Participants attended follow-up meetings and plugged into a Web site designed to support the initiative. More than 500 participants joined together for the effort, which crossed economic, religious and business boundaries.

- The University of Vermont hoped that undergraduates would form their early college friendships around healthy behaviors. A course was created that incorporated peer support skills into the curriculum. Students were organized into groups of three, and 20 minutes of weekly course time was set aside to discuss wellness goals and their peer support. Students submitted a log of their efforts and a final report on their progress.

- Union Pacific Railroad wanted to create a wellness culture throughout its multi-state network. The company incorporated peer support lessons into Wellness Mentor training for safety captains. Participants were encouraged to serve as wellness mentors, and a referral system was set up for employees seeking assistance with health behavior change.

- A state school system incorporated peer support skills into its health risk appraisal (HRA). Employees checked a box at the end of their online HRA to indicate their desire to be matched with Wellness Coaches. A Web site assisted school employees in working with their Wellness Coaches to lower health risks.

Bringing on the Wellness Revolution Checklist

The following checklist helps determine how you might continue to work with *Healthy Habits, Helpful Friends*. Consider these approaches to bringing on the wellness revolution:

☐ I explore interests in wellness and will learn more about what is being done to promote wellness in my area as well as nationally.

☐ I explore new knowledge and skills on the relationship between social connections and healing.

☐ I explore new knowledge and skills related to the link between social capital and business outcomes.

☐ I explore new knowledge and skills related to how my community and society benefit from human connections.

☐ I find ways to promote wellness-related peer support in workplaces, groups and organizations.

☐ I join with others in learning more about and improving upon the concept of offering peer support for wellness.

Recommended Books

Aldana, S. G. (2005). *The Culprit & the Cure.* **Mapleton, UT: Maple Mountain Press.**

Dr. Aldana has organized the U.S. evidence linking health to health behavior. The book explains the tragic health consequences of a population that is trending toward unhealthy behaviors. It offers guidance useful for examining personal practices and for setting behavior change goals.

Allen, J. (2008). *Wellness Leadership.* **Burlington, VT: Healthyculture.com.**

Wellness Leadership is a guidebook for creating a workplace culture that supports healthy lifestyles. It is a guidebook for managers, supervisors, wellness committees and other wellness champions. The book focuses on four skills: (1) creating a shared wellness vision, (2) serving as an effective role model, (3) aligning cultural influences with wellness, and (4) monitoring and celebrating success. It includes case stories, assessment tools and checklists. The Wellness Leadership approach was first developed for Fortune 500 companies such as Johnson & Johnson and Union Pacific Railroad. It is now being used in hundreds of businesses, schools and communities globally.

Ardell, D. B. (2007). *Under the Influence of a Wellness Lifestyle.* **Duluth, MN: Whole Person Associates.**

Dr. Ardell is best known for his wit and wisdom in explaining how the wellness approach differs from the traditional approach to health and illness. This book explains how we would all benefit from adopting wellness lifestyles. *Under the Influence* features 69 tips for aging healthfully, with panache and the highest possible quality of life. Dr. Ardell's monthly and weekly insights are also available in *The Ardell Wellness Report* at www.seekwellness.com/wellness.

Bandura, A. (1976). *Social Learning Theory*. Englewood Cliffs, NJ: Prentice-Hall.

Albert Bandura is best known for his research on modeling behavior. This book includes a discussion of the role of modeling in shaping behavior.

Cohen, D. & Prusak, L. (2001). *In Good Company*. Boston, MA: Harvard Business School Press.

Good social relationships make for good business. These authors have compiled extensive evidence for how social bonds, referred to as social capital, not only increase teamwork, but are essential to good customer relations and even to the vitality of entire industries. They show how the breakdown of social capital leads to complications such as the need for increased paperwork and litigation.

Harris, T. A. (1973). *I'm OK – You're OK*. New York, NY: Avon Books.

James, M. & Jongeward, D. (1996). *Born to Win*. Reading, MA: Addison-Wesley.

These two books explain transactional analysis, a method of examining the hidden messages in our conversations with others. For example, there is a tendency for conversations about lifestyle to be experienced as being between a parent and a child. Do we come across as adults, children or parents? Peers can use transactional analysis to untangle confusing conversations. Generally speaking, you will want to transform the conversation so that everyone feels like an adult.

Huang, C. A. & Lynch, J. (1995). *Mentoring: The Tao of Giving and Receiving Wisdom*. San Francisco, CA: HarperCollins.

This book offers a Taoist philosophy perspective on mentoring. A short list of words such as *trustfulness* and *decisiveness* are used to discuss the mentoring process.

Leutzinger, J. & Harris, J. (2006). *How & Why People Change Health Behavior.* **Omaha, NE: Health Improvement Solutions.**

This book shares health behavior change success stories. These stories are inspiring and offer insight into the many ways people give and get help with lifestyle change.

Lipman, D. (1995). *The Storytelling Coach.* **Little Rock, AR: August House.**

This book goes beyond teaching readers how to help people tell stories. *The Storytelling Coach* provides important principles for supporting others.

Marlatt, G. A. & Gordon, J. R. (2005). *Relapse Prevention.* **New York, NY: Guilford Press.**

This book provides an extensive review of the research on relapse and offers recommendations for helping people to keep their lifestyle change efforts on track.

Maslow, A. H. (1968). *Toward a Psychology of Being.* **Second Edition. New York, NY: D. Van Nostrand Company.**

This book tells important truths about human potential and motivation. Maslow explains the hierarchy of human needs. The hierarchy of motivation begins with basic survival. At the other end of his continuum is a vision of full mental health, called self-actualization. Using Maslow's framework, we can begin to understand individual values and beliefs. We can use this knowledge to help people better achieve their full potential.

Ornish, D. (1998). *Love & Survival.* **New York, NY: Harper Collins.**

Dr. Ornish assembles the massive evidence that our relationships hold the key to whether we get sick, when we die and how fast we recover from illness. The book discusses a broad range of studies that show that the quality of our communities, our participation in those communities and how we relate to each other plays a powerful role in health that is at least as important as other risk factors such as smoking and inactivity.

Ornish, D. (1990). *Dr. Dean Ornish's Program for Reversing Heart Disease.* **New York, NY: Random House.**

Dr. Ornish has been brilliant at proving to a skeptical medical community that adopting a healthy lifestyle can reverse heart disease. Participants in Ornish's programs maintain their behaviors through support groups and by distancing themselves from common, but unhealthy, cultural norms. We can learn a lot from the achievements of program participants.

Ornstein, R. & Sobel, D. (1989). *Healthy Pleasures.* **Reading, MA: Addison-Wesley.**

Ornstein and Sobel provide compelling evidence that nearly everything that people naturally like to do is good for them. Sex, touching, eating, smelling, laughing, and seeing things of beauty all reduce our risk of getting sick and help us toward a speedy recovery. The authors believe that we pay too much attention to telling people what is risky and not enough attention to what is fun and pleasurable. They give ample justification for putting pleasure back into life. The authors also remind their readers about life's simple pleasures.

Prochaska, J. O., Norcross, J. C. & DiClemente, C. C. (1994). *Changing for Good.* **New York, NY: William Morrow and Company.**

It is normal to view lifestyle change as an event rather than as a process. For example, someone might say, "I quit smoking on July 1, 2006." The authors of *Changing for Good* have found that it is far more helpful to view change as an ongoing process. The primary advantage of working with a process is that it lowers failure rates. In addition, treating lifestyle change as a process makes it possible to work with people who either are not ready to act or are having difficulty sustaining new lifestyle practices. The authors have identified six stages (discussed in this book in Chapter 2, "Setting Behavior Change Goals") that are common to lifestyle change. They explain how we can work the six-stage process to achieve lasting results.

Putnam, J. D. (2000). *Bowling Alone.* New York, NY: Simon & Schuster.

Professor Putnam offers an in-depth look at how social relationships have ebbed and flowed in American life. He points out that we have lost approximately a quarter of our positive social interaction in our homes, at work and in our community. He shows how these trends adversely affect communities, families, democracy, health, business activity and overall quality of life. Robert Putnam examines hundreds of studies that show the negative impact of current trends. He offers guidance in reversing the current breakdown.

Travis, J. W. & Ryan, R. S. (2004). *Wellness Workbook.* Third Edition. Berkeley, CA: Celestial Arts.

Wellness is more than just not being sick. This book broadens and deepens our wellness vision with an examination of the many facets of wellness. The authors see wellness as a process of discovery and growth, and when reading the *Wellness Workbook* you can't help but discover new and relatively unexplored facets of your own life. This book examines all aspects of the human experience, with subjects as diverse as how we communicate, have sex, enjoy music and approach spirituality.

Glossary

Barriers to Change — Successful behavior change frequently requires resources such as time, equipment, mental focus and the cooperation of others. Lack of needed resources makes it difficult to modify behavior and constitutes a barrier to change. You can help your peer in coping with, overcoming and eliminating barriers to change.

Cultural Climate — A sense of community, a shared vision and a positive outlook are social environmental factors that enhance the capacity of individuals and organizations to grow. A sense of community provides for trust and openness. A shared vision enables people to be inspired by a common direction. A positive outlook makes it possible to use individual and collective strengths in meeting challenges. Together, these factors constitute the level of cultural climate that is present at work, at home or in the community. Peer support is frequently directed at limiting exposure to unhealthy social climates and increasing exposure to settings with strong senses of community, shared visions and positive outlooks.

Cultural Norms — The accepted and expected behavior of a culture. Sometimes such behaviors are referred to as "the way we do things around here." People are most likely to be aware of norms when they are new to a culture and are wondering how they are expected to behave. You can help determine if norms at home, at work and in the community support desired healthy behavior. Goals could be set for reducing contact with subcultures that have unsupportive norms. You can also identify groups that have strong norms for desired health behavior. For example, someone seeking to be physically active is likely to benefit from becoming a member of a walking group.

Cultural Touch Points — Subcultures and the broader society influence behavior through broad and overlapping mechanisms called touch points. They are rewards, confrontation, modeling, recruitment and selection, orientation, training, communication, including what is talked about and measured, relationship development, including how people form teams and friendships, rites, rituals and symbols, including holidays, events and important stories, and resource commitment, including how time and money are spent. You examine these touch points to determine how social influences support or fail to support behavior change goals. You work with your peer to find or create subcultures that more fully support desired behavior.

Extrinsic Rewards — Peers, groups and society reinforce behavior through social recognition, benefits, incentives or other forms of payment. These rewards are known as extrinsic because they are provided by others. Prizes, praise, job promotion and salaries are examples of extrinsic rewards. You can provide praise and other extrinsic rewards for progress toward your peer's health behavior change. You may also be helpful in seeking out the extrinsic rewards that may be available for achieving healthy lifestyle goals.

Intrinsic Rewards — Healthy behaviors have varied benefits to the changer. An intrinsic reward is a benefit that directly results from behavior change, for example, feeling more energetic after becoming more fit. An ex-smoker gets fewer colds, a longer life expectancy, improved athletic performance and a reduced risk of becoming impotent (for men). This is over and above the new freedom and lowered expense of breaking free of smoking addiction. You can assist in identifying the many positive rewards that are the direct result of the new health behavior.

Peers — Coworkers, spouses, housemates, friends, neighbors and co-participants in rehabilitation, health or wellness programs have interests and experiences in common. Peers have similar standing and power. Peers are the people in our groups, workplaces and communities that we view as equals. Our peers can play important roles in helping us achieve personal goals.

Relapse — People often revert to previous, undesired practices when attempting to change unhealthy habits. These setbacks are called relapses. Peers help limit relapses by developing strategies for coping with and avoiding difficult situations. When relapse occurs, you assist your peer with getting back on track, limiting his self-doubt and guilt and adjusting change tactics.

Role Model — It's likely that someone has achieved the same behavior change goal your peer seeks under very similar circumstances. A person who has achieved such a change could become a role model if she is willing to tell her story. A lot can be learned from such success experiences. They are proof that change is possible and desirable. Role models can explain what worked and what did not work for them. You do not need to be the role model for your peer. You can help find and interview potential role models.

Stages of Behavior Change — Successful behavior change tends to follow this six-step progression. The first stage of behavior change is devoted to developing the reasons for making the change. Stage two involves picking a time for making the change. The third stage involves selecting the strategies for making the change. Stage four is the action stage when behavior begins to change. Stage five is focused on keeping the new behavior going. The final or sixth stage is a time when the new desired behavior is firmly in place and the person is ready to move on to other goals. You can help to determine where your peer is in the change process so that appropriate goals and tasks can be set. You can also celebrate success along the way and use the stages of behavior change to reestablish progress after any relapse.

Wellness — People can consciously choose to live in ways that maximize their health, quality of life and personal performance. Personal wellness is multidimensional and holistic, encompassing mental and physical well-being as well as a person's relationships with others and nature. You can assist in setting personally satisfying wellness goals that are both positive and affirming.

Wellness Buddies — Sometimes peers partner up to achieve wellness goals. Wellness buddies are friends, family and coworkers who achieve goals together. An example of wellness buddies would be two friends who get together for a morning walk to achieve physical activity goals. New relationships are sometimes formed specifically for companionship in taking on a wellness goal. Such wellness buddy relationships may form in support groups, at health seminars, in rehabilitation programs and at health clubs. You could be a wellness buddy to your peer. Often, however, you can assist in finding another peer interested in becoming his wellness buddy.

Wellness-related Peer Support — Listening and offering words of encouragement are typical forms of support given by friends, family and coworkers to achieve healthy habits. Your support goes beyond such assistance by strategically focusing on a full range of lifestyle change support, including help with setting goals, eliminating barriers to change, identifying role models, locating supportive environments, working through relapse and celebrating success. Follow-through is another distinctive feature of your wellness-related support. You meet regularly with your peer to keep behavior change moving forward.

References

A Call to Kindness

Allen, J. (1984). Correlates of success in lifestyle change efforts. Paper presented at the 92nd annual meeting of the American Psychological Association, Toronto, Canada.

Allen, J. (2001). Building supportive cultural environments. In *Health Promotion in the Workplace*, Michael P. O'Donnell, editor, Third Edition, Delmar Publishers, Inc., Albany, NY, pp. 202-217.

Allen, R. F. & Allen, J. (1983). Lifegain: A new way of helping young people to create positive health supporting cultures. *New Designs for Youth Development*, 4:5; pp. 21 28.

Allen, J. (2002). The role of mentoring in health promotion. *The Art of Health Promotion*. March/April, 6:4; pp. 1-12.

Travis, J. W., & Ryan, R. S. (2004). *Wellness Workbook: How to Achieve Enduring Health and Vitality*. Third Edition. Berkley, CA: Celestial Arts.

Setting Behavior Change Goals

Prochaska, J. O., Norcross, J. C., & DiClemente, C. C. (1994). *Changing for Good: A Revolutionary Six-stage Program for Overcoming Bad Habits and Moving Your Life Positively Forward.* New York, NY: William Morrow and Company.

Identifying Role Models

Bandura, A. (1977). *Social Learning Theory*. Englewood Cliffs, NJ: Prentice-Hall.

Jonas, S. (1996). *The Essential Triathlete*. New York, NY: The Lyons Press.

Working through Relapse

Seligman, M. E. P. (1998). *Learned Optimism*. New York, NY: Pocket Books.

Celebrating Success

Prochaska, J. O., Norcross, J. C., & DiClemente, C. C. (1994). *Changing for Good: A Revolutionary Six-stage Program for Overcoming Bad Habits and Moving Your Life Positively Forward*. New York, NY: William Morrow and Company.

Bringing On the Wellness Revolution

Consumer Reports on Health (2006). August, 18:8; p. 5.

Steve G. Aldana (2005). *The Culprit & the Cure: Why Lifestyle Is the Culprit Behind America's Poor Health and How Transforming That Lifestyle Can Be the Cure*. Mapleton, UT: Maple Mountain Press. Available from Wellness Councils of America at www.welcoa.org.

Ornish, Dean (1997). *Love & Survival: The Scientific Basis for the Healing Power of Intimacy*. New York, NY: HarperCollins.

Depner, C. E., & Ingersoll-Dayton (1988). Supportive relationships in later life. *Psychology and Aging*, 3:348-57 as cited in Dean Ornish (1997), *Love & Survival: The Scientific Basis for the Healing Power of Intimacy*. New York, NY: HarperCollins, p. 29.

Cohen, D., & Prusak, L. (2001). In *Good Company: How Social Capital Makes Organizations Work*. Boston, MA: Harvard Business School Press.

Putnam, R. D. (2000). *Bowling Alone: The Collapse and Revival of American Community*. New York, NY: Simon & Schuster.

Also available from the
Human Resources Institute, LLC

Wellness Leadership: Creating Supportive Environments for Healthier and More Productive Employees empowers managers, wellness committee members and other wellness champions to create a workplace culture that supports healthy lifestyles. Such a culture of health saves lives, cuts medical costs, enhances productivity, improves morale and adds new vitality to work groups. *Wellness Leadership* explains how to create a shared wellness vision, serve as an effective role model, align cultural influences and monitor/celebrate success. Revealing self-tests, a culture survey, information about legal issues, guidelines for establishing wellness committees, leadership stories and checklists take the guesswork out of creating a culture of health. The book also serves as a text for Wellness Leadership Training.

Wellness Leadership was written by Judd Allen, Ph.D. in 2008. It is available from the Human Resources Institute as a paperback and as an audiobook for $14.95. The book can be ordered at www.healthyculture.com. Call (802) 862-8855 to order the audiobook and for information about volume discounts.

Healthy Habits, Helpful Friends
Quick Order Form

Fax orders: 802-862-6389

Telephone orders: Call 800-800-3004 in the U.S. or 802-862-8855

Email orders: Info@healthyculture.com

Postal orders: Healthyculture.com, 151 Dunder Road, Burlington, Vermont, 05401 USA

Number of Books _____

Cost of 1st book $14.95.

Cost of 2nd book $9.95. Call for bulk order pricing.

Please add $5 for first book shipped by air within the U.S. and $2 for each additional book.

Please add 8% sales tax for books shipped to a Vermont address.

Please add $9 for first book shipped outside the U.S and $5 for each additional international order.

Name

Address

Telephone

Email

We gladly accept checks in U.S. funds payable to the Human Resources Institute, LLC

To pay by MasterCard or VISA

Card Number _____

Expiration date _____

Billing address if other than shipping address